Alzheimer's Disease: Clinical Diagnostic and Therapeutic Strategies

Alzheimer's Disease: Clinical Diagnostic and Therapeutic Strategies

Editor: Juan Daniels

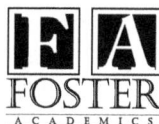

FOSTER
ACADEMICS

www.fosteracademics.com

www.fosteracademics.com

F A
FOSTER
ACADEMICS

Cataloging-in-Publication Data

Alzheimer's disease : clinical diagnostic and therapeutic strategies / edited by Juan Daniels.
    p. cm.
Includes bibliographical references and index.
ISBN 978-1-63242-784-7
1. Alzheimer's disease. 2. Alzheimer's disease--Diagnosis. 3. Alzheimer's disease--Treatment.
4. Alzheimer's disease--Patients--Care. I. Daniels, Juan.
RC523 .A49 2019
616.831--dc23

Foster Academics,
118-35 Queens Blvd., Suite 400,
Forest Hills, NY 11375, USA

ISBN 978-1-63242-784-7 (Hardback)

Contents

Preface

In my initial years as a student, I used to run to the library at every possible instance to grab a book and learn something new. Books were my primary source of knowledge and I would not have come such a long way without all that I learnt from them. Thus, when I was approached to edit this book; I became understandably nostalgic. It was an absolute honor to be considered worthy of guiding the current generation as well as those to come. I put all my knowledge and hard work into making this book most beneficial for its readers.

Alzheimer's disease refers to a chronic neurodegenerative illness which generally starts slowly and worsens over time, and may cause dementia. Dementia includes the brain disorders which cause a gradual but long-term decrease in one's ability to think and remember. Some of the common symptoms of Alzheimer's disease include short-term memory loss, mood swings, disorientation, problems with language and behavioral issues. The causes of Alzheimer's disease are not defined. However, a genetic involvement has been found in most of the cases. Treatment methods include validation therapy, reminiscence therapy, psychotherapy and simulated presence therapy. This book brings forth some of the most innovative concepts and elucidates the unexplored aspects of Alzheimer's disease. The topics included herein on Alzheimer's disease are of utmost significance and bound to provide incredible insights to readers. This book includes contributions of doctors and experts which will provide innovative insights into the diagnosis and therapeutic management of this disease.

I wish to thank my publisher for supporting me at every step. I would also like to thank all the authors who have contributed their researches in this book. I hope this book will be a valuable contribution to the progress of the field.

Editor

The Alzheimer's Patient in the Emergency Department — Specificities of Care

De Breucker Sandra, Pepersack Thierry and
Bier Jean-Christophe

Additional information is available at the end of the chapter

1. Introduction

In Belgium, like in almost all other European countries, Alzheimer's disease affects a growing number of people as our western population is growing older and the life expectancy is expanding.

We estimate the prevalence of AD to 800.000 people in France and 420.000 people in Benelux (Belgium, Netherlands, Luxemburg).

Although the prevalence is very low before age of 70, it exceeds 20 % of men and 30 % of women after 90 years old [1].

Alzheimer's disease has a heavy impact on physical, psychological and social equilibrium of the patient and his family. Alzheimer's disease has still a bad image in the society, because it is described like a slowly progressive but inexorable illness, affecting not only intellectual abilities, but also physical integrity.

Beyond the basic care, the Alzheimer patients need from professionals a specific support, which implies a better knowledge of the illness and listening skills of the patient and his family.

Alzheimer's disease patients need regularly to be hospitalized, and the emergency room is their main way to be admitted to the hospital. However, the lack of knowledge of professionals on Alzheimer's disease induces suffering for the patient and his family, as they are too often considered as heavy and non-cooperating patients.

The purpose of this article is to give some useful bases to inhospital caregivers who are confronted to Alzheimer's disease patients, especially in emergency unit.

2. Alzheimer's disease

Alzheimer's disease is the most frequent cause of dementia, accounting for 50% to 60% of all cases. It is a neurodegenerative disease, which affects cognitive functions, psychological and behavioural balance. Alzheimer's disease is a neurodegenerative disorder in which two proteins (amyloid-β and Tau) undergo pathological changes, consisting in brain accumulation of an insoluble form of amyloid-β, and in hyperphosphorylation of the tau protein with modifications of the stereotactic configuration. Although the exact chronology and interaction between these proteins is still debated, it is generally accepted that these alterations arise years and probably decades before the appearance of any clinical symptoms [2].Thus, physiopathology associated an accumulation of beta amyloid peptides in senile plaques and tangles (induced by tau protein abnormalities) in the neurofibrils with lipid oxidation and peroxidation, glutamatergic toxicity, and on inflammation, leading to neuronal apoptosis. Another physiopathological change concerns

Other physiopathological change concerns possible heavy metals accumulation, vascular or infectious processes... Finally, there is an increasing evidence that vascular dysfunction plays an important role in the clinical decompensating Alzheimer's disease [3].

Its course is slow, insidious and lasts for years.

Psychological and Behavioral Symptoms of Dementia (BPSD) may appear at any time of the disease but usually appear later in its course. They can represent loss of initiative to manage daily activities (apathy), changes in the personality (irritability, paranoiac thoughts, delusions) or changes in the mood and the behaviour (anxiety, depression, aggressiveness, appetite disorders, wandering). Noteworthy, sleep disorders, depression and anxiety or even apathy may all emerge before the onset of cognitive symptoms in many cases.

Finally, the neuronal loss is high and more physical neurological syndromes emerge (epilepsy, walking disorders, higher risk of falls, immobilization, swallowing disturbances, malnutrition and dehydration).

As for many syndromes, the clinical diagnosis is based on different criteria [4,5].

First, the patient's and family 's anamnesis informs the clinician when and how the disease began, how it evolves and if it has a negative impact on daily activities.

The personal and familial history, socio-educational and co-morbid features will complete the history.

Biological tests can be restricted to those allowing to exclude pathologies interfering with cognition, for example folic acid or vitamin B12 deficiency, dysthyroidism, ionic and metabolic disorders. When the clinical features or history suggest syphilis, HIV or borreliosis, specific serologies should be performed.

Cognitive assessment should be completed with a validated screening test, such as a Mini Mental State Examination (MMSE) [4]. Space-time orientation and immediate memory represent 16 points of the total 30 points. In case of doubt, a total score equal or over 24/30 should be followed by a comprehensive cognitive assessment performed by a neuropsychologist. It emphasizes multiple cognitive disorders and helps the clinician to define the diagnosis as best as possible.

Brain neuroimaging (CT scan, magnetic resonance imaging) completes the workup. It detects potentially treatable cerebral lesions (tumors, hematoma, hydrocephaly,...), and associated causes (vascular lesions). It also gives anatomic indices to describe specific Alzheimer features (ie hippocampic atrophy).

Functional neuroimaging (Pet Scan, SPECT) explores topographic hypometabolic zones, helping to approach the diagnosis when clinical features are unusual.

Finally, lumbar puncture is a complementary diagnostic tool, it allows to confirm the diagnosis if the clinical presentation is more atypical: low levels of b-amyloid 42 and high levels of tau and phosphotau protein seem highly sensitive and specific (80%) to Alzheimer's disease.

When the diagnosis is defined, the Alzheimer's disease management should begin with the announcement of the diagnosis to the patient and his family. It is important to take into account the patient's anxiety related to the delay of the disease announcement itself to find the good moment to announce it. Most of Alzheimer patients wish to be informed of their diagnosis (72 to 96% from one study to another) and 7% of caregivers wish their parents to be informed from what they suffer, to respect his/her autonomy of decision [6,7].

The information on the disease must be clear, concise and should focus on the course of illness, its main comorbidities, the need to provide more help for daily activities...

It is also important to talk about medicolegal issues, such as the ability to drive a car, to set up a personal property manager.

The caregiver approach should consist in a specific education on the illness, whether for the basics or a true course called « psychoeducation ». A study demonstrated that a caregiver's specific training delays the time of institutionnalization until 500 days [8], and decreases the risk of caregiver's mood disorders [9]. An American study showed that a daily home caregiver to help the main caregiver lowered the number of hospitalizations, the length of stay of demented patients [10].

The treatment consists in a global approach; pharmacological and non-pharmacological approaches should always coexist.

Two drug classes are currently available; cholinesterase inhibitors (donepezil, rivastigmine, galantamine) and N Methyl D Aspartate receptor antagonists (memantine). Although they have only a minor effect on the course of the illness, cholinesterase inhibitors are actually recommended in mild to moderate Alzheimer's disease.

A French study showed that Alzheimer patients treated by cholinesterase inhibitors are later institutionalized than those not treated [11]. Memantine has a greater protective effect on memory in later stages of the disease, and it seems to have a positive impact on some behavioural disturbances [12,13]. The combination of the two classes is probably promising, further studies are expected to confirm it clearly.

The treatment of behavioural and psychological and social disorders needs to first identify the triggering and/or worsening factors (environmental factors, organic causes such as pain, constipation, infections; iatrogenic causes and depression).

Non-pharmacological approach includes different therapies: aromatherapy, musical therapy, physical exercises… Until now, none of these therapies have been shown effective, due to the lack of reproducible methodology from one study to another [14].

If necessary, neuroleptics can help to manage BPSD, following the rule « the lowest dose, the shortest time » as possible, to avoid adverse reactions (drowsiness, falls, extrapyramidal syndromes) and its bad impact on quality of life, wellness feeling, and the risk to worsen cognitive disorders [15,16].

3. The caregiver's burden

Formal caregivers, (spouses or children), informal caregivers (neighbours, friends, home care nurses) suffer from the « collateral distress » of Alzheimer's disease. This is influenced by the lack of knowledge on the illness, its course and its prognosis. Moreover, caregivers are often the first who refer their proxy to the memory clinic, because they suffer, without knowing why: the feel « abnormally exhausted ». Studies show that caregivers suffer more from anxiety, depression, and alcohol abuse and have a higher risk of mortality [4].

At the diagnosis announcement, different kinds of reactions are observed.

Some of them deny it. Some others tend to be more protective with the patient, and are usually hyperinvesting in the care of their parent.

Sometimes conflicts appear between the patient, his family and the institution of care. It is particularly true if the family feels guilty and ambivalent toward their parent and because they refer the heavy task on care people.

Before the patient will be referred to a nursing home, the main caregiver must be psychologically and physically sustained by a trained team, and he must be informed on the possibilities to have periods of rest during the course of the illness.

Home care should be strictly organised and adapted from the beginning until the end of the course of the disease. Even after the institutionalization, the family should be followed specifically.

Advanced directives for the patient could also be discussed with them.

Though defined as a chronic disease, the disease progression to terminal illness is rarely recognized as a « palliative process ». An American study followed 300 institutionalized Alzheimer's patients and their proxies during 18 months. 55% of the patients died during this period; 41% had pneumonia, 52% had fever episode, 85% had problems to eat alone. In emergencies, 46% had dyspnea, 39% experienced pain. In the last 3 months of life, 40% had experienced « aggressive therapies »: they were hospitalized; they were referred to an emergency department, or even underwent artificial nutrition.

When patients and their proxies had been well informed on the prognosis and the course of the disease, patients had a more worthy end-of-life experience [17]. It emphasizes the importance to educate the care staff, whether for home care, hospital care or nursing home care [18].

4. The patient with dementia at the emergency department

Among patients older than 60 years old admitted in emergency department, 13% have cognitive disorders. When they are admitted at hospital by another way, only 8% have cognitive problems [19].

Most of time, the urgent admission of a demented patient is more justified by the lack of structural or human support than the acute illness itself: the emergency room becomes the only « wipe out » for burden families, sometimes also for burden professionals in nursing homes.

More, literature reports that proxies express very few their wish to find an alternative structure to take care of their parents [20].

The reason of admission is most often a somatic problem.

In a prospective study conducted by B Vellas et al, the two first causes of admission of demented patients in emergency wards were behavioural disorders (26,3%) and falls (18,6%) [21].

A retrospective study in United Kingdom, between 2002 and 2007, showed that demented patients (20% Alzheimer, 11% vascular dementia, 69% not defined in the medical file) were more frequently admitted via the emergency room than non-demented patients. The diagnosis of dementia is rarely evoked in the file (6-10%). Most are hospitalized for somatic problems (syncope, pneumonia, urinary tract infection, dehydration) and more significantly than non-demented patients [22].

In a French study (REAL.FR), investigators followed 516 patients with light to moderate Alzheimer disease during one year. 27% of them were hospitalized at least once. Predictive factors of hospitalization were: caregiver's burden (the most frequent), loss of autonomy in one or more basic daily activities (Katz scale) or in two or more instrumental daily activities, the presence of at least 2 current illnesses, depressive disorders, polypharmacy, disinhibition, delirium, score > 5 on Reisberg's illness rating scale (moderate dementia or severe cognitive decline) and the need for external help for housekeeping [23]. After 2 years of follow-up, predictive factors of rehospitalisation were need for basic daily activities, caregiver's burden and high level of BPSD based on NPI scale (Neuropsychiatric Inventory) [24].

In case of real emergency, the GP should refer the patient with a detailed file containing medical and dementia history, current medications, and a brief summary of home care providers' journal, to distinguish chronic and new symptoms. For example, alteration of vigilance is a challenging situation with a broad differential diagnosis: an underlying acute medical illness, epilepsy, drug intoxication, delirium should always be excluded.

It is important to note that most of common pathologies associated with advancing dementia have an underlying illness that needs a specific causal treatment.

Bradshaw et al studied 250 patients aged over 70 with a co-morbid mental health problem and followed them up for 180 days. Twenty-seven per cent did not return to their original place of residence after the hospital admission, and 31% had died after 180 days. Significant predictors for poor outcomes were co-morbidity, nutrition, *cognitive function, behavioural and psychiatric problems and depression* [25].

Medical doctors working in the emergency unit should avoid the use of neuroleptics, or other sedative drugs to treat delirium and BPSD, and a non-pharmacological approach should always be proposed. This implies that any new problematic symptom, including agitation, delirium, paranoia, hallucination, and anxiety … should preferably be managed in collaboration with the physicians who know the patient and the course of the disease. A conservative and comprehensive management of the probable cause of the problem (loss of senses such as sight or hearing; changing habits or care behaviour,..) is the most appropriate.

When drug will be offered, causal effect treatment with the fewest side effects is preferred. It is particularly important to pay attention to any anticholinergic effects and to possible interactions with other medications.

In all cases, we should also exclude organic cause (metabolic disorder, including urinary infections, subdural hematoma in case of fall or even the occurrence of new epilepsy...) before considering the appropriate treatment.

4.1. Delirium and dementia

Delirium is very common in elderly patients admitted in the emergency unit. Risk of delirium is higher for demented patients. It is sometimes the first symptom leading to the diagnosis of dementia.

Most of the time, causes of delirium are not purely neurological and toxic, metabolic causes (hypoglycemia, anemia, heart failure), drugs interactions, current infections or pain have all to be tracked.

Features of delirium are characterized by altered vigilance status, cognitive disorders not related to previous cognitive state, symptoms of rapid onset and fluctuation and a strong evidence of underlying organic disease (DSM IV-TR) [26]. Demented patients with delirium are less able to explain their symptoms than non-demented patients and than demented patients without delirium. They have more difficulties to understand explanations and diagnosis delivered by professionals in the emergency ward [27]. Moreover, delirium in urgent situations is a prognostic factor for loss of autonomy: according to a study of Vida, delirious patients loose more autonomy than non-delirious patients [28]. Finally, delirium is an independent prognostic factor for length of stay and risk of mortality at 6 months [29,30]. In the absence of altered mental status, this syndrome might be missed unless it is actively looked for using a validated delirium assessment.

The environment of the emergency room is seldom adapted to patients with delirium: people have to wait several hours to be managed, rooms have no windows, there is no time markers in the rooms (no clocks, diaries), meals are served at every hours night and day.

It is therefore important to screen for delirium: the most used screening is CAM (Confusion Assessment Method) [31]. Health care providers in emergency units have often not enough time to assess completely the situation, to communicate efficiently with the patients and to take care of their needs.

In front of patient with acute or subacute delirium; fluent aphasia has to be excluded. It could be interpreted as confusion. If the onset of aphasia was sudden, brain imagery and electroencephalogram should always be done.

Management of delirium involves ensuring safety, improving functioning, identifying and treating the illness underlying the delirium, and use of antipsychotics or benzodiazepines to control behavioural symptoms and prevent mortality. Haloperidol, an old typical neuroleptic is the most commonly used antipsychotic in delirium. Atypical antipsychotics may be as efficacious as haloperidol in the treatment of delirium, but have less side effects [32]. In addition, to restore good quality of sleep and normal circadian rhythm, the use of melatonin can sometimes help. Anticholinesterases or memantine have few impacts on delirium in emergency cases [33]. However, their chronic prescription could decrease the risk of delirium and BPSD in dementia especially in case of Alzheimer disease.

Non pharmacological approach in emergency units would consist in faster management of the patient in quiet rooms with windows, clocks and calendars should be implemented. Beds with barriers, with comfortable mattress should be proposed.

4.2. Paranoia and dementia

Paranoia is a manifestation induced by excess of dopaminergic metabolites. As for other delirious ideas, it can also results from errors of interpretation or of reasoning, especially in dementia (objects lost interpreted as stolen...) [34].

In combination with a decrease of dopaminergic drugs, a conservative treatment has first to be considered. Anticholinesterase and memantine have both a top-grade places to avoid as far as possible the use of neuroleptics in terms of side effects, particularly in case of dementia [35-37]. Sometimes, trazodone 50 to 200 mg/day can help [38].

However, in emergency and only during the acute phase, haloperidol 1 to 4 mg could be proposed. But, in case of chronic use, new generation of neuroleptics (quetiapine for example) should be preferred with the necessity to track any extrapyramidal signs and to adapt the treatment very regularly.

4.3. Depression and dementia

Depression is frequently associated with dementia either as a triggering factor of the disease or as its consequence. However, depression is rarely the cause of emergency admission in case of dementia. If suicidal risk should be systematically screened, its arisen is exceptional perhaps as a consequence of memory disturbances, mood and cognitive fluctuations. Planning and executive difficulties could also explain the low rate of suicide in demented patients. Impulsive suicidal acts are nevertheless possible. Depression influences cognitive and functional capacities of all individuals, demented or not. This is of particular importance in case of minor and major neurocognitive deterioration, and it should be systematically screened and treated, in order to improve the quality of life of the patient and its caregivers, and to preserve the patient's residual functional and cognitive capacities. The preferential choice will then consider a drug with as least as possible interactions with other concomitant medications (often a selective serotonin reuptake inhibitor), taking into account the impact on appetite and sleep of the patient. A recent meta-analysis showed that psychological interventions associated with antidépressive drugs can reduce symptoms of depression and clinician-rated anxiety for people with dementia [39].

On the other hand, any caregiver's depression should be aggressively pursued and handled in view of its great incidence and of its heavy impact.

Nevertheless, we can't underestimate the ability of emergency caregivers to communicate with demented patients: Eder points out their need of knowledge of dementia, ie the different kinds of dementia, its progression, its symptoms, in order to communicate and manage adequately these patients [40].

Restraint is also a frequent ethical problem in emergency units. It raises ethical questions to all of us but especially to caregivers: « Should I respect the patient's autonomy, if he is in danger for himself or for others? How to justify it? » [41].

Finally, the length of stay in emergency unit depends on the downstream bed availability. Time spent by caregivers to find a bed is also wasted time to communicate with the patient.

Therefore, the management of these patients must be lead by an interdisciplinary approach. Nevertheless, in some countries like France, only 20% of hospitals have a geriatric unit. There is then an urgent need to sensitize medical hospital managers and policy makers to improve the geriatric offer in terms of acute settings.

At a medical level, the emergency physician should work together with geriatricians to understand how to integrate the acute illness into the patient's geriatric syndromes.

It is therefore useful to define a care pathway for the demented patient, from home care to hospital management.

We could imagine to apply to emergency units what already exists in terms of technological innovation for home care of elderly (demented) patients: for example, the European HOPE project (Smart Home for Elderly People) aimed to improve communication and information to proxies to take care of their elderly demented parent; this system helped to maintain quality of life, and to improve health care, security and communication with the patient [42].

5. Proposition of a care pathway of demented patients

The general practitioner (GP) is the first health care provider involved [20]. He should be trained to inform families of the dementia's symptoms, their expected evolution and their potential complications. This is first, to prevent crisis and proxy's burden.

A crisis is an episode of acute disorganization with symptoms that lead patients and their caregivers to call an emergency care help. It refers to a sudden change in the course of the patient's and family's habits, while it is very important to maintain them stable for dementia's stability [43].

It happens too often that patients are admitted to emergency units on the request of GP, without evident urgent situation. When the problem is not urgent, the GP should refer the demented patient to geriatric or neurological consultation, or to the geriatric day hospital.

We developed in Belgium a specific care program for the geriatric patient which could offer alternative approach for the demented patient: since 2007, Belgian hospitals had to develop pilot projects for geriatric day hospitals, internal liaison (mobile team for geriatric patients hospitalized in other units than geriatric departments) and external liaison with home care and nursing home care providers. The referring GP contacts the coordinator of the geriatric care program and they decide together when and how to admit the patient at hospital, in order to avoid the mandatory passage to the emergency department if the patient doesn't require urgent care. It allows also providing counselling on how to adapt transiently home care.

6. Conclusion

Alzheimer's disease is a frequent pathology. It would be considered as a pandemic illness in the future 20 years. As the demented patient is often admitted at hospital by the emergency unit, it is crucial that emergency caregivers have the best knowledge of the disease, to offer the best adapted care, to support family and to avoid unnecessary admissions.

Acknowledgements

The authors report no conflict of interest for this manuscript.

In addition to the authors, we thank Mrs Micheline Burg and Mrs Christel Cleutinx for their careful review of the English version of the manuscript.

Author details

De Breucker Sandra[1*], Pepersack Thierry[1] and Bier Jean-Christophe[2]

*Address all correspondence to: Sandra.De.Breucker@erasme.ulb.ac.be

1 Erasme University Hospital– Free University of Brussels, Department of Geriatrics, Brussels, Belgium

2 Erasme University Hospital– Free University of Brussels, Department of Neurology, Brussels

References

[1] Lobo A, Launer LJ, Fratiglioni L, Andersen K, Di Carlo A, Breteler MM, Copeland JR, Dartigues JF, Jagger C, Martinez-Lage J, Soininen H, Hofman A. Prevalence of dementia and major subtypes in Europe: A collaborative study of population-based cohorts. Neurologic Diseases in the Elderly Research Group. Neurology. 2000;54(11 Suppl 5):S4-9.

[2] Jack CR Jr, Albert MS, Knopman DS *et al* (2011). Introduction to the recommendations from the National Institute on Aging–Alzheimer's Association workgroups on diagnostic guidelines for Alzheimer's disease. Alzheimers Dement; 7: 257–62

[3] Iadecola C. The overlap between neurodegenerative and vascular factors in the pathogenesis of dementia. Acta Neuropathol. 2010 Sep;120(3):287-96.

[4] Hort J, O'Brien JT, Gainotti G, Pirttila T, Popescu BO, Rektorova I, Sorbi S, Scheltens P; on Behalf of the EFNS Scientist Panel on Dementia. EFNS guidelines for the diagnosis and management of Alzheimer's disease. Eur J Neurol. 2010 ; 17:1236-1248.

[5] American Psychiatric Association-DSM IV. Manuel diagnostique et statistique des troubles mentaux. Paris : Masson, 1996.

[6] Johnson, H. & Bouman, W. P. & Pinner, G. (2000) On disclosing the diagnosis in Alzheimer's disease: a pilot study of current attitudes and practice. International Psychogeriatrics 2000 ; 2(2) : 221-9.

[7] Pinner G. Truth-telling and the diagnosis of dementia. British Journal of Psychiatry 2000 ; 176 : 514-515.

[8] Mittelman MS, Haley WE, Clay OJ, Roth DL. Improving caregiver well-being delays nursing home placement of patients with Alzheimer disease. Neurology 2006; 67: 1592–1599.

[9] Mittelman MS, Brodaty H, Wallen AS, Burns A. A three-country randomized controlled trial of a psycho-social intervention for caregivers combined with pharmacologi-

cal treatment for patients with Alzheimer disease: effects on caregiver depression. Am J Geriatr Psychiatry 2008; 16: 893–904.

[10] Shelton P, Schraeder C, Dworak D, Fraser C, Sager MA. Caregivers' utilization of health services: results from the Medicare Alzheimer's Disease Demonstration, Illinois site. J Am Geriatr Soc. 2001;49(12):1600-5.

[11] Gillette-Guyonnet S, Andrieu S, Cortes F, Nourhashemi F, Cantet C, Ousset PJ, Reynish E, Grandjean H, Vellas B. Outcome of Alzheimer's disease: potential impact of cholinesterase inhibitors. J Gerontol A Biol Sci Med Sci. 2006;61(5):516-20.

[12] Becker M, Andel R, Rohrer L, Banks SM. The effect of cholinesterase inhibitors on risk of nursing home placement among medicaid beneficiaries with dementia. Alzheimer Dis Assoc Disord. 2006 Jul-Sep;20(3):147-52.

[13] Gauthier S, Loft H, Cummings J. Improvement in behavioural symptoms in patients with moderate to severe Alzheimer's disease by memantine: a pooled data analysis. Int J Geriatr Psychiatry 2008; 23: 537–545.

[14] Douglas S, James I, Ballard C. Non-pharmacological interventions in dementia. Advances in Psychiatric Treatment 2004 ;10: 171-179.

[15] Ballard, C. G., O'Brien, J., James, I., et al. Dementia: Management of Behavioural and Psychological Symptoms. Oxford: Oxford University Press ; 2001.

[16] McShane, R., Keene, J., Gedling, K., et al. Do neuroleptic drugs hasten cognitive decline in dementia? Prospective study with necropsy follow-up. BMJ 1997 ; 314 : 211–212.

[17] Mitchell SL, Teno JM, Kiely DK, Shaffer ML, Jones RN, Prigerson HG, Volicer L, Givens JL, Hamel MB. The clinical course of advanced dementia. N Engl J Med. 2009 Oct 15;361(16):1529-38.

[18] Villars H, Oustric S, Andrieu S, Baeyens JP, Bernabei R, Brodaty H, Brummel-Smith K, Celafu C, Chappell N, Fitten J, Frisoni G, Froelich L, Guerin O, Gold G, Holmerova I, Iliffe S, Lukas A, Melis R, Morley JE, Nies H, Nourhashemi F, Petermans J, Ribera Casado J, Rubenstein L, Salva A, Sieber C, Sinclair A, Schindler R, Stephan E, Wong RY, Vellas B. The primary care physician and Alzheimer's disease: an international position paper. J Nutr Health Aging. 2010 ;14(2):110-20.

[19] Shah MN, Jones CM, Richardson TM, Conwell Y, Katz P, Schneider SM. Prevalence of depression and cognitive impairment in older adult emergency medical services patients. Prehosp Emerg Care. 2011;15(1):4-11.

[20] Moulias R, Hervy MP, Ollivet C, Emmanuelli X. Alzheimer et maladies apparentées : traiter, soigner et accompagner au quotidien. Paris : Elsevier Masson ; 2005.

[21] Nourhashémi F, Andrieu S, Sastres N, Ducassé JL, Lauque D, Sinclair AJ, Albarède JL, Vellas BJ. Descriptive analysis of emergency hospital admissions of patients with Alzheimer disease. Alzheimer Dis Assoc Disord. 2001;15(1):21-5.

[22] Natalwala A, Potluri R, Uppal H, Heun R. Reasons for hospital admissions in dementia patients in Birmingham, UK, during 2002-2007. Dement Geriatr Cogn Disord. 2008;26(6):499-505.

[23] Balardy L, Voisin T, Cantet C, Vellas B. Predictive factors of emergency hospitalisation in Alzheimer's patients: results of one-year follow-up in the REAL.FR Cohort. J Nutr Health Aging. 2005;9(2):112-6.

[24] Voisin T, Andrieu S, Cantet C, Vellas. Predictive factors of hospitalizations in Alzheimer's disease: a two-year prospective study in 686 patients of the REAL.FR study. BJ Nutr Health Aging. 2010;14(4):288-91.

[25] Bradshaw LE1, Goldberg SE, Lewis SA, Whittamore K, Gladman JR, Jones RG, Harwood RH. Six-month outcomes following an emergency hospital admission for older adults with co-morbid mental health problems indicate complexity of care needs. Age Ageing. 2013 Sep;42(5):582-8.

[26] American Psychiatric Association. Diagnostic and Statistical Manual of Mental Disorders (IV-TR). 4th-Text Revised. Washington, D.C. : Arlington ; 2000.

[27] Han JH, Bryce SN, Ely EW, Kripalani S, Morandi A, Shintani A, Jackson JC, Storrow AB, Dittus RS, Schnelle J. The effect of cognitive impairment on the accuracy of the presenting complaint and discharge instruction comprehension in older emergency department patients. Ann Emerg Med. 2011 Jun;57(6):662-671.

[28] Vida S, Galbaud du Fort G, Kakuma R, Arsenault L, Platt RW, Wolfson CM. An 18-month prospective cohort study of functional outcome of delirium in elderly patients: activities of daily living. Int Psychogeriatr. 2006;18(4):681-700.

[29] Han JH, Shintani A, Eden S, Morandi A, Solberg LM, Schnelle J, Dittus RS, Storrow AB, Ely EW. Delirium in the emergency department: an independent predictor of death within 6 months. Ann Emerg Med. 2010 Sep;56(3):244-252.

[30] Han JH, Eden S, Shintani A, Morandi A, Schnelle J, Dittus RS, Storrow AB, Ely EW. Delirium in older emergency department patients is an independent predictor of hospital length of stay. Acad Emerg Med 2011 ; 18 : 451-7.

[31] Monette J, Galbaud du Fort G, Fung SH, Massoud F, Moride Y, Arsenault L, Afilalo M. Evaluation of the Confusion Assessment Method (CAM) as a screening tool for delirium in the emergency room. MGen Hosp Psychiatry. 2001;23(1):20-5.

[32] Grover S, Matoo SK, Gupta N. Usefulness of atypical antipsychotics and choline esterase inhibitors in delirium: a review. Pharmacopsychiatry. 2011;44(2):43-54.

[33] Overshott R, Karim S, Burns A. Cholinesterase inhibitors for delirium. Cochrane Database Syst Rev. 2008; (1):CD005317.

[34] Perez-Madriñan G1, Cook SE, Saxton JA, Miyahara S, Lopez OL, Kaufer DI, Aizenstein HJ, DeKosky ST, Sweet RA. Alzheimer disease with psychosis: excess cognitive impairment is restricted to the misidentification subtype. Am J Geriatr Psychiatry. 2004;12(5):449-56.

[35] Campbell N, Ayub A, Boustani MA, Fox C, Farlow M, Maidment I, Howards R. Impact of cholinesterase inhibitors on behavioral and psychological symptoms of Alzheimer's disease: a meta-analysis. Ann Pharmacother. 2008 Jan;42(1):32-8.

[36] Maidment ID, Fox CG, Boustani M, Rodriguez J, Brown RC, Katona CL. Efficacy of memantine on behavioral and psychological symptoms related to dementia: a systematic meta-analysis.Clin Interv Aging. 2008;3(4):719-28.

[37] Daiello LA1, Beier MT, Hoffmann VP, Kennedy JS. Pharmacotherapy of behavioral and psychological symptoms of dementia: a review of atypical antipsychotics. Consult Pharm. 2003 Feb;18(2):138-52, 155-7.

[38] López-Pousa S1, Garre-Olmo J, Vilalta-Franch J, Turon-Estrada A, Pericot-Nierga I. Trazodone for Alzheimer's disease: a naturalistic follow-up study. Arch Gerontol Geriatr. 2008 Sep-Oct;47(2):207-15.

[39] Orgeta V1, Qazi A, Spector AE, Orrell M. Psychological treatments for depression and anxiety in dementia and mild cognitive impairment. Cochrane Database Syst Rev. 2014; 22;1:CD009125.

[40] Eder S. The Alzheimer's challenge. Emerg Med Serv. 2005;34(6):99-103.

[41] McBrien B. Exercising restraint: clinical, legal and ethical considerations for the patient with Alzheimer's disease. Accid Emerg Nurs. 2007;15(2):94-100.

[42] Pilotto A, D'Onofrio G, Benelli E, Zanesco A, Cabello A, Margelí MC, Wanche-Politis S, Seferis K, Sancarlo D, Kilias D. Information and communication technology systems to improve quality of life and safety of Alzheimer's disease patients: a multicenter international survey. J Alzheimers Dis. 2011;23(1):131-41.

[43] Michon A. Crisis intervention in dementia. Psychol Neuropsychiatr Vieil. 2006;4(2): 121-5.

2

Lipids and Lipoproteins in Alzheimer's Disease

Sophie Stukas, Iva Kulic, Shahab Zareyan and
Cheryl L. Wellington

Additional information is available at the end of the chapter

1. Introduction

Cholesterol is a key structural component of the brain, and cholesterol transport and distribution within the central nervous system (CNS) is mediated by a lipid metabolic cycle that includes generation of apolipoproteins as lipid carriers, lipidation by cholesterol and phospholipid transporters, enzyme remodeling of these particles and their receptor-mediated uptake and turnover in cells. It is becoming increasingly appreciated that Alzheimer's Disease (AD) patients often have comorbid conditions such as cardiovascular disease, type II diabetes mellitus, or hypertension, each of which can greatly affect lipoprotein metabolism, especially at the vessel wall and thereby possibly contribute to AD pathogenesis. Here we review the known biology of lipids and lipoproteins in the CNS and discuss how alterations in lipid metabolism may impact AD pathogenesis. Apolipoprotein E (*APOE*) is the best established genetic risk factor for AD and the major apolipoprotein expressed in the brain. In addition, genome-wide association studies (GWAS) have identified several other genes associated with AD risk that function in lipid or lipoprotein metabolism, including clusterin (*CLU*), ATP binding cassette (ABC) transporter A7 (*ABCA7*), and apoE receptors. Understanding how lipid/lipoprotein metabolism in the brain and body affect cognitive function may therefore offer new insights in developing more effective therapeutic approaches for dementia.

2. Lipid and lipoprotein metabolism in the CNS

2.1. General biology and function of lipids and lipoproteins in the CNS

The brain is the most cholesterol-rich organ in the body, with an average cholesterol content of 15-20 mg/g wet weight compared to 2 mg/g for peripheral tissues in the adult mouse [1].

The majority of the brain's sterol content is located in free cholesterol, 70-80% of which is in myelin. Cholesterol, sphingomyelin and phospholipids form the major structural components of cellular membranes, with cholesterol, phosphatidylcholine and phosphatidylethanolamine being the most abundant lipids in synaptic vesicles [2]. Many lipids also participate in important signaling pathways in the brain, with lipid-mediated second messengers derived from sphingomyelin and phosphatidylinositol, activation of G- protein coupled receptors and nuclear receptor activation being particularly important [1, 3].

Name	Major Sites of Production in the Brain	Main Functions in Healthy Brain	Potential Role in AD

ApoE	• Astrocytes
	• Microglia
		• Lipid transport
		• Aβ homeostasis
		• BBB integrity
		• Cerebrovascular health
		• Innate immune response
		• Reelin signaling
			• Involved in Aβ metabolism: deposition, transport across the BBB, clearance through ISF and the CSF pathways, and enzymatic degradation
			• Regulation of inflammation
			• ApoE4, the most established AD genetic risk factor, is associated with:
			    1. Impaired Aβ degradation and clearance
			    2. Increased tau phosphorylation and formation of NFT
			    3. Ineffective lipid transport
			    4. Impaired synaptic integrity
			    5. Reduced ability to suppress inflammation

Clusterin	• Astrocytes • Choroid plexus epithelial cells • Neurons	• Golgi chaperone • Inflammatory response • Complement regulation • Cell Cycle regulation • Reelin signaling	• Third most highly associated susceptibility locus for AD. • Potentially involved in Aβ sequestration, degradation and clearance
ApoA-I	• Not produced in the brain	• Reverse cholesterol transport • Vascular endothelial health	• AD comorbidities such as type II diabetes and hypercholesterolemia lead to apoA-I dysfunction • Reduction of CAA, neuroinflammation, and oxidative stress in mouse models of AD

Table 1. Major Apolipoproteins in the Brain

As lipids are insoluble in aqueous environments, neutral lipids are transported through bodily fluids on lipoprotein particles consisting of amphipathic apolipoproteins that surround and stabilize their lipid cargo. The general structure of mature spherical lipoproteins consists of a core of neutral cholesterol ester and triglycerides surrounded by amphipathic free cholesterol and phospholipids at the exposed surface, all of which are encapsulated by apolipoproteins

[3]. Four major lipoprotein classes, defined by their buoyant density, are found in the circulation: high density lipoproteins (HDL), low density lipoproteins (LDL), very low density lipoproteins (VLDL) and chylomicrons. While LDL, VLDL and chylomicrons are triglyceride rich, HDL is triglyceride poor, and the HDL-like lipoprotein species found within the CNS contain even less triglyceride than plasma HDL. As apolipoprotein B (apoB), the major apolipoprotein of chylomicrons, VLDL, and LDL, is not found in the CNS, lipoprotein metabolism in the brain and cerebrospinal fluid (CSF) is based entirely on a lipoprotein class that most resembles plasma HDL with respect to size, shape, and density [4-11]. In rodents, astrocytes secrete apoE-containing lipoproteins that are primarily composed of phospholipids (~6 µg/ml) and cholesterol (~13 µg/ml), 0-18% of which is found in the esterified form. These nascent lipoprotein particles are discoidal, ranging from 9-17 nm in diameter with a density of 1.00-1.12 g/ml [7, 10]. Clusterin, also known as apolipoprotein J (apoJ), is also produced by astrocytes but is secreted virtually free of lipids [7, 10, 12]. Conversely, whereas lipoprotein particles found in CSF are of a similar diameter (11-20 nm) and density (1.063-1.12 g/ml) to those secreted by astrocytes, they are distinguished by their spherical shape and a greater proportion of phospholipids and cholesterol, with approximately 70% of cholesterol found as cholesterol esters [5, 7, 8, 10, 13]. ApoE and apolipoprotein A-I (apoA-I) are the major apolipoproteins present in CSF by mass, with apolipoproteins A-II, A-IV, D, CI, CIII, and clusterin also present to a lesser extent [5, 8-11]. In the healthy CNS, lipoproteins regulate the transport, delivery and distribution of lipids. In addition, lipoproteins are also thought to regulate many functions in the CNS including inflammation, oxidative stress, vascular tone, cerebral blood flow, and blood brain barrier (BBB) integrity (Table 1) [14].

2.2. Apolipoproteins present in the CNS

ApoE is present at 2-10 µg/ml in human and mouse CSF [8, 13, 15, 16] and at 10-50 ng/ml in interstitial fluid (ISF) from both wild-type mice as well as in targeted replacement mice that express human apoE [17]. ApoE is the most abundant apolipoprotein expressed within the brain, where it is synthesized and secreted by astrocytes and, to a lesser extent, microglia [5]. Secreted apoE particles are lipid-rich, containing equal amounts of apoE and lipid, and carry cholesterol secreted by astrocytes [10, 18]. Indeed, lipidation of apoE is essential for its stability and function [19-21]. Humans express three *APOE* isoforms that differ from one another by two amino acid residues; *APOE2* (cys112, cys158), *APOE3* (cys112, arg158) and *APOE4* (arg112, arg158), with the *APOE3* allele being the most common and the *APOE2* allele being the least frequent in the general population [19]. The resulting apoE2, apoE3 and apoE4 proteins therefore have both structural differences with respect to protein folding as well as functional interactions with respect to their ability to bind to lipids and apoE receptors [22]. In addition to mediating cholesterol transport to neurons, apoE has other functions in the brain such as regulating vascular health and the innate immune system (Table 1) [23].

Brain tissue has one of the highest concentrations of clusterin, which is expressed in astrocytes, epithelial cells of the choroid plexus, and selected neuronal subsets [24]. As a result, clusterin is present in CSF at concentrations of 4-6.5 µg/ml in healthy human adults [25]. In humans, due to the presence of three alternative mRNA start sites, the clusterin gene *CLU* is expressed as three transcriptional isoforms. At the protein level, clusterin exists in two major forms: a 50 kDa nuclear form and a 75-80 kDa glycosylated secreted form [26]. Although clusterin is best known for its role as a chaperone, it also appears to be involved in the inflammatory response and complement regulation, the cell cycle, and endocrine functions (Table 1) [27].

Unlike apoE and clusterin, apoA-I is not expressed in either murine or human brain [28-31], suggesting that its presence in the CNS reflects transport across the BBB and/or the blood-CSF-barrier (BCSFB) following its production from hepatocytes and enterocytes. Although *in vitro* experiments suggest that apoA-I can transcytose across cultured endothelial cells [32], an *in vivo* study shows that peripherally injected apoA-I rapidly localizes to choroid plexus epithelial cells with negligible association in cerebrovascular endothelial cells, suggesting that peripherally derived apoA-I may gain access to the CNS primarily by crossing the BCSFB [31]. The concentration of apoA-I in CSF is ~3-4 µg/mL, or 0.26% of plasma levels, in humans [8, 13, 15, 33] and 0.02 µg/mL, or 0.01% of plasma levels, in wild-type mice [31]. The physiological functions of apoA-I in the CNS are not well understood but are hypothesized to be similar to those of CNS apoE (Table 1) [14].

In addition to apoE, clusterin, and apoA-I, other apolipoproteins are also detected in the CNS, including apoD, apoC-I, apoC-III, apoA-II, and apoA-IV [8, 9, 11], each of which is detected in human CSF [5, 8-11]. It has been shown that apoD, an apolipoprotein with antioxidant and anti-inflammatory properties, is produced in neuroglial cells, pia mater cells, and perivascular cells in the human brain [34, 35].

2.3. Cholesterol and Phospholipid Transporters

Lipid-poor apolipoproteins receive cholesterol and phospholipids from membrane bound transporters that are part of the ABC transporter family. The ubiquitously expressed transporter ABCA1 mediates the transfer of cellular cholesterol and phospholipids from cellular membranes to lipid-poor apolipoprotein acceptors including apoA-I and apoE [36- 39], a process that is essential for the production of both plasma and CSF HDL. HDL plays a critical role in the regulation of lipid homeostasis, and is particularly important for cells such as macrophages and microglia that form part of the innate immune system. ABCA1 activity in these phagocytic cells is exquisitely sensitive to cholesterol accumulation, and by catalyzing efflux of excess cholesterol and phospholipids to apoA-I and apoE acceptors, ABCA1 activity helps to maintain intracellular cholesterol balance. In humans, mutations that block ABCA1 function cause Tangier Disease, which is characterized by a 95% loss of plasma HDL cholesterol and apoA-I levels due to rapid catabolism of lipid-poor apoA-I by the kidney. ABCA1-dependent lipidation of CNS apoE is also critical for its stability as both total body and brain-specific loss of ABCA1 in mice leads to a significant 60-80% reduction of brain and CSF apoE [20, 21, 30]. Whether ABCA1 also regulates apoE levels in the brain of Tangier Disease patients is not known. Notably, Wahrle et al. did not observe significant differences in CSF apoE levels between control subjects versus those with ten different *ABCA1* single nucleotide polymorphisms (SNPs), suggesting that these SNPs may not have a significant effect on human ABCA1 function in the CNS [16]. In mice, total body deletion of ABCA1 results in a significant and proportional reduction of apoA-I levels by 60-90% in plasma, brain tissue and CSF [40].

Intriguingly, brain-specific deletion of ABCA1 in mice leads to a significant increase of apoA-I protein levels in brain tissue and CSF [30]. The mechanisms that regulate the distribution of apoA-I between peripheral and CNS compartments remain to be fully determined.

Highly homologous to ABCA1, ABCA7 is also abundantly expressed in microglia, oligodendrocytes, neurons, and astrocytes in both humans [41] and mice [42, 43]. Although the potential for ABCA7 to act as a cholesterol and/or phospholipid transporter in the CNS is unknown, when overexpressed in human embryonic kidney cells, ABCA7 can mediate the transfer of phospholipids and sphingomyelin, but not cholesterol, to lipid-poor apoA-I and apoE [42]. The relative contribution of ABCA7 to the *in vivo* generation of plasma HDL cholesterol appears to be minimal and may be influenced by sex, as decreases in plasma total cholesterol and HDL cholesterol are only detected in female *Abca7-/-* mice [43]. Instead, ABCA7 may be more involved is modulating the phagocytic activity of macrophages, particularly following injury or infection; whether this is also true in brain microglia will be important to address in the future [44, 45]. One critical difference between ABCA1 and ABCA7 is the distinct manner in which they are regulated by cholesterol. Whereas ABCA1 expression is induced by activation of the Liver-X-Receptor (LXR) pathway in response to increased cellular cholesterol content, ABCA7 induction is unaffected [42, 43]. Instead, ABCA7 expression is primarily regulated by sterol regulatory element binding protein 2 (SREBP-2) and is thus repressed in cholesterol-laden cells [44].

Following initial lipidation, nascent HDL lipoproteins can receive additional lipids from the cholesterol transporters ABCG1 and ABCG4 [46], which are abundantly expressed in grey and white matter of the brain [47]. Unlike ABCG4, whose expression appears to be restricted to neurons, astrocytes, and the retina, ABCG1 is widely expressed throughout the body and is found in the liver, intestine, lungs, kidney and spleen in addition to neurons, astrocytes, microglia, and choroid plexus epithelial cells [47, 48]. In addition to lipid efflux activity, ABCG1 and ABCG4 are also believed to regulate intracellular transport of cholesterol and sterols and vesicle trafficking in the brain [47, 48].

2.4. Enzymes involved in lipoprotein metabolism

Many enzymes involved in lipoprotein metabolism are found in CSF, although for most, their CNS expression patterns and functional roles have not been explored to the same extent as in the periphery. For example, lecithin cholesterol acyltransferase (LCAT), phospholipid transfer protein (PLTP), and cholesteryl ester transfer protein (CETP) are all detectable in brain tissue and CSF [13, 49-53] and, as they have established roles in plasma lipoprotein metabolism, it is of interest to understand whether they function similarly in the brain.

In plasma, LCAT is the enzyme responsible for generating the cholesterol ester core characteristic of mature circulating lipoproteins, including HDL. As the more hydrophobic cholesterol esters migrate to the core of the lipoprotein particle, the discoidal nascent particle takes on its mature spherical shape. LCAT-mediated esterification of cholesterol serves not only to generate mature HDL particles, but also to maintain the downward cholesterol gradient between the cell and the lipoprotein particle, enabling further cholesterol efflux [54]. LCAT is present in human CSF at levels corresponding to 2.2-2.5% of that in serum and migrates with γ-like lipoproteins [13, 49]. In mice, LCAT is secreted mainly by astrocytes, can be activated by both apoA-I and apoE, and esterifies free cholesterol contained on glial-derived apoE-containing lipoproteins [55]. LCAT may therefore play a role in maturation of discoidal lipoprotein particles secreted from glia to the spherical particles that circulate in CSF by catalyzing the cholesterol esterification of immature CNS lipoprotein particles [5, 7, 56].

PLTP is another enzyme intimately involved in the maturation and turnover of lipoprotein particles within the circulation and CNS. PLTP's primary activity involves the transfer of phospholipids between HDL particles, thus modulating HDL size and composition, and transferring lipids between apoB-containing lipoproprotein particles and HDL [53]. Within the CNS, PLTP is highly expressed by neurons, astrocytes, microglia, oligodendrocytes, BBB endothelial cells, choroid plexus ependymal cells and can be found both in brain tissue and CSF in human and animals [57-61]. Within CSF, PLTP is associated with apoE-containing lipoproteins where it actively participates in phospholipid transport [13, 62, 63] with activity corresponding to 15% of plasma levels in humans [62] and 23% of plasma levels in rabbits [59]. Functionally, PLTP has been reported to regulate apoE expression and secretion by astrocytes [63] and participate in neuronal cell signalling [64].

In plasma, CETP catalyses the bi-directional transfer of cholesterol esters from HDL in exchange for triglycerides from VLDL and LDL, thereby reducing circulating HDL concentration and increasing its size [65]. CETP can potentially diffuse through the BCSFB and enter the brain from plasma. However, it is not clear whether CETP is produced in the brain. Yamada et al. reported CETP-like immunoreactivity in astrocytes in healthy human brain [51]. Albers et al. have suggested that CETP is locally produced in the brain, as they were able to detect CETP in human CSF samples at concentrations higher than what would be expected from simple diffusion of proteins across the BCSFB [66]. However, Demeester et al. were unable to detect CETP in human CSF and CETP mRNA in the human brain [13]. A few other studies have also not detected CETP mRNA in the CNS of rabbits and cynomolgus monkeys [59, 67]. Undoubtedly, more research on the production and the role of CETP in the CNS of healthy individuals is needed.

2.5. Receptors involved in lipoprotein uptake and turnover

Lipoprotein uptake and delivery of lipids into target cells of the CNS is regulated by the low density lipoprotein receptor (LDLR) family [68]. The four major apoE receptors in the CNS are LDLR, lipoprotein receptor related protein-1 (LRP1), very low density lipoprotein receptor (VLDLR), and apolipoprotein E receptor 2 (apoER2) [69]. Of these, LDLR is the only receptor that has apoE as its only known ligand in the CNS [69]. LDLR and LRP1 levels are inversely correlated with brain apoE levels as deletion or overexpression of these receptors in mice increases or decreases brain apoE levels, respectively [70-73]. VLDLR and apoER2 also serve as essential receptors for the neuromodulatory ligand Reelin, which is involved in long term potentiation, learning and memory [74-76]. Like apoE, clusterin can also bind to VLDLR and apoER2 to regulate Reelin signaling (Table 1) [77]. LDLR, LRP1, VLDLR and apoER2 are all expressed on neurons, which have a high LRP1:LDLR ratio. LRP1 and LDLR are also found on astrocytes, which have a low LRP1:LDLR ratio, and LRP1 and VLDLR are found on microglia [78-81]. Solubilized forms of these receptors, generated via ectodomain shedding or splice variants lacking the transmembrane domain, possibly contribute to negative feedback and inhibition of lipoprotein uptake [82]. Of note, the lipoprotein related protein 2 (LRP2), also known as megalin, and the neuronal sortilin- related receptor (SORL1 receptor) are also additional apoE receptors expressed in the CNS [83, 84].

3. Alterations to lipids and lipoproteins in Alzheimer's disease

The neuropathology of AD is defined by the presence of amyloid plaques and neurofibrillary tangles (NTFs), which are composed of deposited amyloid-beta (Aβ) peptides and filamentous hyperphosphorylated tau, respectively [85]. In addition to parenchymal amyloid plaques, most AD patients also have accumulation of amyloid in cerebral blood vessels, known as cerebral amyloid angiopathy (CAA) [14, 86]. Furthermore, neuronal degeneration and dysfunction, the brains of AD patients are often marked by significant signs of chronic inflammation, oxidative stress and vascular dysfunction. Not surprisingly, apolipoproteins, the lipids they carry, and the transporters responsible for their lipidation may be intimately involved in each step of the disease. In particular, the interrelationship between cerebrovascular dysfunction and AD is increasingly appreciated. Epidemiological, clinical, neuropathological and pathophysiological evidence shows that several cardiovascular risk factors also increase AD risk, including age, sex, hypertension, dyslipidemia, and type II diabetes [87-90]. Dementia progresses more rapidly in patients with cerebral infarcts [90- 93] and infarction and other forms of brain injury may potentiate AD pathophysiology [94- 96]. Importantly, many of these cardiovascular risk factors include aspects of dysfunctional lipid and lipoprotein metabolism, which likely occurs at the vessel wall. However, compared to the wealth of knowledge about lipid and lipoprotein physiology in large peripheral vessels, little is known about the mechanisms by which vascular risk factors for AD may impair the function of cerebral vessels. Importantly, BBB dysfunction may contribute to inflammatory processes in the CNS, where exacerbated inflammatory responses or failure to resolve inflammatory reactions are increasingly recognized to play important roles in AD pathogenesis [97].

3.1. Changes in brain lipid composition and their direct effects in AD

One often overlooked neuropathological observation initially reported by Alois Alzheimer is the presence of adipose inclusions in the brain, which Alzheimer defined as "extraordinarily strong accumulation of lipoid material in the ganglion cells, glia and vascular wall cells, and the particularly numerous fibril-forming glia cells in the cortex and, indeed, in the entire central nervous system" [98]. Almost all major classes of lipids have some correlation with AD pathogenesis [99]. A recent review by Kosicek and Hecimovic reported that the *post-mortem* brain levels of phosphatidylinositol, phosphatidylethanolamine, ethanolamine plasmalogen, and sulfatide are decreased in AD, while the levels of ceramide are increased [100]. Though not as extensively studied, it has been reported that CSF levels of ceramide are increased, while the levels of sulfatide are decreased in AD [101, 102]. Furthermore, studies by Soderberg et al. and Tully et al. report lower levels of n-3 and n-6 polyunsaturated fatty acids, which are major components of phospholipids, in AD brain compared to healthy controls [103, 104]. Changes to the levels of these lipid classes affects not only the structural properties of the membranes, but also numerous signaling and trafficking pathways that are heavily involved in the normal functioning of the cells in the CNS [99, 105].

Changes to CNS lipid composition can also influence the production of Aβ peptides. As the generation of these peptides involves several lipid-associated steps, including intracellular trafficking and inter-membrane proteolytic cleavage, it is not surprising that, in addition to genetic changes that alter Aβ production, there are also indirect, lipid- dependent changes that can affect production of Aβ. Aβ peptides are derived via sequential proteolytic processing of the amyloid precursor protein (APP) by β-secretase and γ- secretase. This leads to liberation of Aβ peptides 38-46 amino acids in length into the extracellular space [106-108]. Of these, Aβ40 and Aβ42 are quantitatively the most important for amyloid deposition [109]. In healthy brains, the vast majority of APP is processed by α-secretase, followed by γ-secretase cleavage, which prevents toxic Aβ peptide generation [110]. All of the enzymes involved in APP processing are transmembrane proteins, raising the hypothesis that the lipid composition and lipid organization in the membrane may affect Aβ production [111]. Numerous *in vitro* studies have focused on determining the role of specific lipid classes in APP processing. For example, it has been shown that reducing membrane cholesterol lowers the levels and activity of β-secretase and reduces γ- secretase activity, decreasing Aβ production [99, 112]. Altered cholesterol content in lipid rafts, regions in the cellular membrane enriched with cholesterol and sphingolipids, affects the localization of enzymes involved in Aβ production, which can lead to changes in amyloidogenic APP processing [99]. Moreover, sphingolipids have been reported to regulate γ-secretase activity [99, 113, 114]. Interestingly, expression of familial presenilin (PS) mutations, which are mutations in components of the γ-secretase complex, affects sphingolipid metabolism, suggesting an interplay of genetics and lipid metabolism in the context of APP processing. Furthermore, *in vitro* elevation of ceramide, which is composed of sphingosine and fatty acids, increases β-secretase stability and promotes Aβ biogenesis [115].

The production of Aβ peptides is not unique to AD pathology, but a constitutive process that is a product of normal cell metabolism throughout life, confirmed by its secretion from primary cells in culture and its presence in the plasma and CSF of healthy individuals [108, 116, 117]. Therefore, it is possible that disrupted Aβ homeostasis, either via increased production or impaired degradation and clearance, leads to its net accumulation in the brain, triggering subsequent neurotoxicity. Aβ production is clearly enhanced in cases of familial early onset AD (<60 years of age), which account for 2-3% of the AD population [118]. In contrast to familial early-onset AD cases, the vast majority of AD subjects who develop cognitive impairment in late life have no genetically-determined net increase in Aβ production. For these late-onset AD patients, who account for up to 99% of the AD population [119], aging, environmental factors, or other genetic-related impairments in Aβ degradation and clearance are thought to lead to the net accumulation of Aβ within the CNS [120-122].

3.2. Apolipoproteins and AD pathogenesis

Of the apolipoproteins present in the CNS, *APOE* has the most established genetic association with AD, influencing the risk, progression, and pathology of the disease (Table 1). The *APOE4* allele is a robust risk factor for late-onset AD and is found in 40-60% of AD subjects depending on ethnicity (the prevalence is lower in Asian compared to Northern European populations) even though its carrier frequency in the human population is approximately 15-20% [123-125]. *APOE4* increases AD risk by 3-fold when inherited in a single copy and greater than 9-fold in homozygous individuals. *APOE4* also accelerates the age of onset of AD [123, 126, 127]. A wealth of pre-clinical and clinical evidence has demonstrated that *APOE4* is associated with earlier and more extensive Aβ and amyloid deposition, which is currently believed to result from a net impairment of Aβ degradation and clearance from the CNS [120, 128]. ApoE affects Aβ metabolism through multiple mechanisms, including transport of Aβ across the BBB, modulation of interstitial fluid (ISF) and CSF clearance pathways, effects on BBB integrity, and modulating the growth of Aβ oligomers and fibrils [129, 130]. Some studies suggest that the risk and severity of CAA is also increased in *APOE4* carriers [131, 132]. Intriguingly, a patient with an ablative mutation in *APOE* was recently described to have no detectable impairment in cognitive, neurological and retinal function, with normal levels of CSF Aβ and tau despite very high plasma cholesterol levels [133], suggesting that apoE may have non-essential functions in the human brain and eye. This observation reflects the prediction made from *Apoe*-deficient mice, which also have greatly increased plasma cholesterol levels and exhibit greatly reduced Aβ retention in the CNS [134-137].

In addition to modulating Aβ, apoE may also be involved in tau phosphorylation. In neurons, hyperphosphorylation of the microtubule-associated protein tau by kinases, including GSK-3β and CDK5, causes the dissociation and aggregation of tau to ultimately form neuro-fibrillary tangles [138]. Under conditions of stress or injury, neurons have been reported to synthesize and process apoE4 to produce neurotoxic C-terminal fragments. Release of these fragments into the neuronal cytosol has been reported to enhance tau phosphorylation and formation of NFT-like structures [139, 140].

ApoE4 has additional deleterious consequences. Compared to apoE3, apoE4 is less effective at mediating cholesterol transport in the brain; human knock-in *APOE4* homozygous mice show reduced total cholesterol and phospholipids compared to wild type mice [81, 141]. The *APOE4* allele has also been implicated in impaired synaptic integrity, as human *APOE4* transgenic mice show lower levels of excitatory synaptic activity that declines to levels comparable to *Apoe* knockout mice by 7 months of age [142]. ApoE4 has also been reported to reduce apoER2 expression at the neuronal surface, impairing the ability of Reelin to enhance synaptic glutamate receptor activity [143].

ApoE plays an integral role in inflammatory processes in the brain. Inflammation of the brain's glial supporting cells, known as neuroinflammation, is a prominent feature AD [144] and contributes to neuronal damage. In response to Aβ or lipopolysaccharide (LPS), LRP1-mediated glial cell activation increases apoE, which can limit the inflammatory response by signaling though LDL receptors to suppress c-Jun N-terminal kinase signaling [145, 146]. There is also evidence that isoform-specific apoE modulation of the innate immune response can modulate Aβ deposition [147]. Consistent with apoE having an anti- inflammatory role, *Apoe*-deficient mice have elevated proinflammatory cytokines in the liver [148]. Importantly, isoform specific effects appear to determine the extent of cytokine induction and may also modulate progression and resolution of CNS inflammation. In mice, apoE4 has reduced ability to suppress the inflammatory response induced by LPS treatment [149] and in the EFAD model (5 familial AD mutations in the presence of human *APOE*), microglial activation in response to Aβ is augmented by the *APOE4* genotype [150]. Indeed, *Apoe*-deficient mice show a similar activation of the inflammatory response to human *APOE4* knock-in mice following LPS injection, implying that apoE4 may lack the anti- inflammatory functions of the other apoE isoforms [151]. Consistent with these findings, non- steroidal anti-inflammatory drugs are associated with a reduced risk of AD only in participants with an *APOE4* allele [152].

According to the AlzGene database, *CLU* is the third most highly associated susceptibility locus for AD following *APOE* and bridging integrator 1 (*BIN1*) (www.alzgene.org). In 2009, two independent GWAS studies identified the C allele of the rs11136000 SNP in the *CLU* gene, which occurs in 88% of Caucasians, to confer a modest risk of AD development (odds ratio (OR) 1.16), whereas inheritance of the T allele is protective (OR 0.86) in Caucasians [153, 154]. Although these findings have been replicated in, and confirmed for, Caucasians of European ancestry, the association of *CLU* polymorphisms and AD risk has not been replicated in African-American, Hispanic, or Arab populations [27, 155]. Since this discovery, estensive work has been conducted in an attempt to delineate the mechanism(s) by which the rs11136000 SNP confers AD risk. Inheritance of the TT versus TC versus CC allele appears to result in either no change [156, 157] or a very subtle 8% decrease [158] of plasma clusterin levels in AD and mild cognitive impairment (MCI) patients, with small 10-17% decreases of plasma clusterin observed in cognitively normal aged-matched controls with the TT allele [156, 158]. Despite minimal effects on circulating clusterin levels with the T allele, inheritance of the C allele of the rs11136000 SNP is associated with both structural and functional changes in the CNS. In young (aged 20-30 years) cognitively normal adults, each copy of the C allele of the rs11136000 SNP is associated with lower white matter integrity [159], decreased coupling and connectivity between the hippocampus and prefrontal cortex during memory processing tasks [160], and neural hyperactivity under emotional working paradigms [161], indicative of early structural and functional abnormalities that may leave the brain more vulnerable to disease during aging. In the elderly, independent of dementia status, the CC allele is significantly associated with longitudinal increases in ventricular volume over a 2 year period [162], and increased resting regional cerebral blood flow in the hippocampus and right anterior cingulate cortex, regions which are important for memory function and default mode network activity, over an 8-year period [163]. Further, the protective T allele is associated with a reduced rate of conversion from MCI to AD (OR 0.25) [164], while the detrimental C allele is correlated with a significantly faster rate of decline in verbal but not visual memory performance in MCI and AD patients [163]. Lastly, with respect to CSF biomarkers, the *CLU* C allele is associated with significantly lower CSF Aβ42 in a Finnish [165] but not American cohort [166], with no association found for either total or phosphorylated tau.

Although the specific mechanisms by which an individual SNP in *CLU* may confer disease risk are not well understood, there are well recognized global changes to clusterin mRNA and protein expression both in the plasma and CNS that are associated with AD pathology and clinical presentation [27]. In non-demented elderly controls and patients with subjective memory complaints, CSF clusterin is positively associated with CSF total and phosphorylated tau [167] and an elevated atrophy rate in the entorhinal cortex of older non- demented adults with low CSF Aβ42 [168]. Whereas older studies did not detect significant differences in CSF clusterin between cognitively normal aged matched controls and AD subjects [25, 169], newer studies that utilize higher sensitivity methods have reported up to a 25% increase of CSF clusterin in AD subjects [170, 171], suggesting that increased CNS clusterin may be detrimental. Within brain tissue, clusterin mRNA is increased after correcting for neuronal loss [172, 173], whereas protein levels are reportedly increased by 40-180% depending on the brain region [172, 174-177]. Within the AD brain, clusterin strongly co-stains with dystrophic neurites, neuropil threads, and intracellular NFT [176, 178, 179], with minimal to moderate co-localization observed with mature amyloid plaques [176, 178, 180, 181] and cerebrovascular amyloid [180]. Unlike the CNS, multiple studies have detected no difference between plasma clusterin levels in non-demented controls, MCI, and AD subjects [157, 182-185]. However, increased baseline plasma clusterin levels are suggestive of increased prevalence and severity of AD pathology and presentation, including brain atrophy, amyloid deposition and worsened cognitive function, with a more rapid clinical progression [186-188].

A mechanistic involvement of clusterin in AD pathology is also supported by *in vivo* preclinical studies (Table 1) [27]. Clusterin appears to be directly involved in neuronal health and Aβ metabolism via a variety of mechanisms. In transgenic AD mice, genetic ablation of clusterin results in a reduction of mature fibrillar amyloid deposits and the dystrophic neurites that are associated with them [189]. Supporting this, a recent study found that co- incubation of Aβ with clusterin leads to a 60% decrease in oligomeric and 42% decrease in fibrillar Aβ binding and uptake by primary microglia, and a 72% reduction in binding and uptake of oligomeric Aβ by primary astrocytes, suggesting that clusterin can impede Aβ degradation by local glia [190]. *In vitro* and *in vivo*, clusterin may also mediate Aβ toxicity and tau phosphorylation via dickkopf-1-driven induction of the Wnt-PCP-JNK pathway [191]. In contrast, other studies have found a beneficial role of clusterin in facilitating Aβ clearance across the BBB via LRP-2 [192] and binding to and sequestering Aβ oligomers, thereby reducing their potential toxicity [193]. Clusterin also participates in various aspects of cell signaling. *In vitro*, clusterin signals via Reelin by binding to apoER2 and VLDLR thereby increasing cell proliferation and neuroblast chain formation in the subventricular zone [77]. Clearly, more research is necessary to fully understand the pathways by which clusterin is involved in brain function and the pathogenesis of AD.

Although apoA-I is relatively abundant in CSF and brain tissue, the physiological roles of apoA-I containing lipoprotein particles in the CNS, their potential influence on AD risk and pathology, and whether they affect AD pathogenesis through actions from one or both sides of the BBB remains unknown [14]. The most established data regarding apoA-I and AD are human epidemiological studies examining the interaction between serum apoA-I and HDL-cholesterol levels with AD risk (Table 1). At mid-life, high serum apoA-I levels resulted in a significantly lower risk (hazard ratio (HR) 0.25) of dementia later in life, [194] while high levels of serum HDL cholesterol (> 55 mg/dL) in cognitively normal elderly was associated with a significantly reduced risk (HR 0.4) of AD even after adjusting for *APOE* genotype and vascular risk factors such as heart disease, diabetes, obesity, hypertension, and lipid lowering treatment [195]. Recently, Reed et al. demonstrated that low plasma HDL cholesterol and apoA-I were associated with and predicted higher amyloid Pittsburgh compound B binding independent of *APOE4* in cognitively normal and MCI elderly subjects [196]. There also appears to be a consistent 20-30% reduction in serum apoA-I in late-onset AD subjects compared to age-matched controls [197-199], with levels of serum apoA-I positively correlating to cognitive function [199, 200]. Further, in symptomatic AD patients, plasma apoA-I levels are negatively correlated with measures of brain atrophy, including hippocampal and whole brain volume and mean entorhinal thickness [186]. Alterations to CSF apoA-I are less clear, potentially due to the small number of studies or sample size, whereas two studies reported a decrease of CSF apoA-I in AD subjects [15, 201], two other studies reported no change [13, 202]. Prospective studies designed and powered to assess the levels, and perhaps more importantly, the function of both plasma and CSF apoA-I-HDL with respect to AD onset and progression are needed to determine if apoA-I-HDL potentially contributes to AD pathology.

Although questions remain about the importance of apoA-I to AD in humans, studies in preclinical AD mouse models support a role for apoA-I in removing amyloid selectively from the cerebral vasculature, leading to reduced neuroinflammation and maintenance of cognitive function (Table 1). Specifically, genetic loss of *Apoa1* is associated with increased CAA, greater inflammation, and exacerbated cognitive impairment, whereas transgenic overexpression of human *APOA1* from its endogenous promoter (driving expression from only hepatocytes and enterocytes) prevented AD-related cognitive decline and reduced both CAA and glial activation in symptomatic APP/PS1 mice [203, 204]. Given the known roles of apoA-I-containing HDL in regulating vascular endothelial health, reducing inflammation and oxidative stress, coupled with the relative contributions of these pathologies to AD, it will be paramount to fully elucidate the function of apoA-I in the CNS and evaluate its therapeutic potential [14].

Although the roles of other CNS apolipoproteins in AD pathogenesis are not as extensively studied, apoD, apoC-I, apoA-IV, and apoC-III may play a role. The most significant change due to aging is observed in gene expression levels of *APOD* [205]; CSF and hippocampal apoD are elevated in AD [206] and correlated with disease severity [207]. ApoC-I colocalizes with Aβ plaques in human AD brain [208] and apoC-I has been suggested to influence neuroin-flammation in AD [209]. The *APOC1* gene is also considered as an AD susceptibility locus, as the H2 polymorphism of *APOCI* is in linkage disequilibrium with *APOE4* [209-211]. Further-more, heterozygosity of the *APOA4* (360:His) allele is more common in AD patients [212]. In APP transgenic mice, *Apoa4* deficiency increases Aβ load, enhances neuronal loss, accelerates cognitive dysfunction and increases mortality [213]. Lastly, apoC-III has recently been reported to be associated with Aβ levels in the periphery and is of possible interest for use as an early biomarker for AD [214].

3.3. Cholesterol and phospholipid transporters in AD

There is a growing body of pre-clinical and clinical evidence that supports the involvement of ABCA1, and recently ABCA7, in the pathogenesis of AD [215]. In mice, ABCA1-mediated lipidation of apoE correlates with a net increase in Aβ clearance [216]. For example, total body deficiency of *Abca1* markedly decreases soluble apoE and increases amyloid plaque-associated insoluble apoE, decreases plasma and CSF apoA-I, and increases Aβ deposits in both paren-chymal and vascular compartments, with no net change in APP production or processing [217-220]. Recently, Fitz et al. demonstrated that haploinsufficiency of *Abca1* significantly exacerbated cognitive deficits, increased Aβ and amyloid deposits, and reduced Aβ clearance in ISF of *APOE4* but not *APOE3* APP/PS1 *Abca1*-/+ mice, suggesting a particularly deleterious state of poorly-lipidated apoE4 compared to apoE3 [221]. Of interest, the presence of apoE4 with *Abca1* hemizygosity leads to a modest but statistically significant decrease in CNS apoE (~10%), decreased CNS and plasma apoA-I by approximately 50 and 20%, respectively, and decreased plasma Aβ42 and HDL cholesterol, with a strong inverse correlation between plasma HDL cholesterol levels and amyloid burden [221]. Both genetic and pharmacological approaches that increase brain ABCA1 activity also increase functional CNS apoE [40, 222] and improve learning and memory with [222-227] or without [228-232] changes in Aβ and/or amyloid burden. Importantly, ABCA1 was required to observe an improvement in cognitive function in APP/PS1 mice treated with the LXR agonist GW3965, suggesting that ABCA1 lipidation of lipid-poor apolipoproteins is essential for cognitive function [229]. It is important to note, however, that these manipulations will affect ABCA1-mediated lipidation of apoE in the brain as well as ABCA1-mediated lipidation of apoA-I in the periphery and potentially the CNS, of which the relative contributions are unknown.

The association of *ABCA1* genetic variants and AD risk in human subjects is not as clear despite more than a dozen studies [216]. In 2013, a meta-analysis was conducted on 13 independent studies totaling 6034 controls and 6214 AD patients that examined whether the *ABCA1* variants R219K rs2230806, I883M rs4149313 and R1587K rs2230808 were associated with AD risk. No significant association was found even after adjusting by ethnicity and sample size [233]. This is consistent with *ABCA1* failing to appear in GWAS [216]. It is important to note, however, that most of the *ABCA1* gene variants in heterozygous patients translate to a relatively small reduction in plasma HDL cholesterol that may or may not increase the relative risk of ischemic heart disease [234, 235], raising the caveat that these variants may not be severe enough to impact brain physiology. As Tangier Disease, in which patients completely lack functional ABCA1, is extremely rare and most patients die before 70 years of age, it is not known whether human ABCA1 deficiency is associated with neuropathological changes relevant to AD [236].

In contrast to ABCA1, numerous independent GWAS have identified associations be-tween multiple *ABCA7* SNPs and AD risk [237-244]. ABCA7 expression has been report-ed to be increased in the brains of AD subjects, with the magnitude of the increase correlating with greater cognitive decline [239, 241]. In 2011, the first two major SNPs of *ABCA7*, rs2764650 [244] and rs3752246 [237], were associated with increased risk of late-onset AD. Two subsequent GWAS found that the rs2764650 SNP was significantly associated with increased neuritic plaque burden [242, 243]. However, both Larch et al. and Vasquez et al. found that the minor allele of the rs2764650 SNP conferred protection from AD by delaying onset and decreasing disease duration, despite increased ABCA7 expression, whereas another study found that rs2764650 neither altered ABCA7 expression or AD risk [238]. In African Americans, the *ABCA7* rs115550680 SNP was shown to increase AD risk by 1.79 even after adjusting for *APOE* genotype, which itself conferred a relative risk of 2.31 [240]. With more *ABCA7* SNPs identified by GWAS to confer AD risk [238], it will be increasingly important to identify the functional consequences of *ABCA7* polymorphisms. In transgenic APP mice, total body loss of *Abca7* increases hippocampal Aβ and amyloid burden with no changes in APP processing or brain levels of ABCA1, apoE, LDLR, or markers of neurodegeneration or synaptic loss [245]. However, increased Aβ and amyloid did not significantly impair any measure of cognitive function, including spatial memory, object recognition, short-term recognition, or fear conditioning [245]. Intriguingly, bone marrow derived macrophages obtained from *Abca7-/-* mice displayed a 50% reduction in Aβ uptake compared to wild type controls, suggesting that phagocytosis may be compromised; however, there were no change to either the number or distribution of microglia or macrophages within the brain parenchyma in AD *Abca7-/-* mice [245].

Despite high expression in the brain, ABCG1 does not appear to have a marked role in AD pathogenesis, as ABCG1 overexpression in AD mice does not significantly change Aβ or amyloid burden [246]. Although a recent GWAS study reported that *ABCG1* SNPs were correlated with neuritic plaque burden in AD subjects [243], the relative risk of *ABCG1* variants has yet to be confirmed.

3.4. LCAT, PLTP and CETP in AD

Although better characterized with respect to their involvement in atherosclerosis, research is emerging regarding the potential role of the lipoprotein modifying enzymes LCAT, PLTP and CETP in AD [53, 65, 247]. One early study in a small group of symptomatic AD patients suggested that CSF LCAT activity was reduced by 50% compared to cognitively normal age-matched controls [13], raising the possibility that aging may influence LCAT activity or LCAT activity may influence AD pathogenesis. Stukas et al. recently tested this hypothesis in mice and found that the abundance and activity of LCAT in liver, cortex and plasma is unaltered by aging or the presence of amyloid deposits [14]. Furthermore, total loss of *Lcat* does not impact apoE levels or lipidation, or Aβ or amyloid metabolism in symptomatic APP/PS1 mice, despite a 70-90% decrease in circulating and CNS levels of apoA-I [14]. These results suggest that CNS lipoproteins need not be in a mature spherical form containing cholesterol esters to participate normally in Aβ metabolism.

PLTP may also be involved in the pathogenesis of AD. Intriguingly, whereas PLTP synthesis by neurons and glia is increased in the early stages of AD [62], its levels, and more importantly, its activity are reduced in brain tissue and CSF of AD patients in later stages [57, 63]. In mice, deletion of *Pltp* increases cerebral oxidative stress, elevates Aβ42, reduces synaptophysin expression, increases BBB permeability and decreases expression of tight junction proteins under basal conditions [61, 248]. Further, intracerebroventricular injection of an oligomeric Aβ peptide leads to exacerbated cognitive impairment in *Pltp-/-* mice compared to wild-type controls [248]. In aged *Pltp-/-* mice, enhanced cognitive impairment is accompanied by increased cortical Aβ42, APP expression, and both β- and γ-secretase activity with decreases in cortical Aβ40 and apoE [249]. These preclinical studies suggest a role for PLTP not only in phospholipid transport, but Aβ homeostasis, neuronal function, barrier integrity, and oxidative stress.

Another enzyme that plays a central role in lipid homeostasis that can potentially affect dementia outcome is CETP. As reduced CETP activity in humans is associated with reduced cardiovascular disease risk, the functions of CETP in atherosclerosis and the potential of CETP inhibitors for cardiovascular disease have been of intense interest [65]. The *CETP* 405V allele, which results in low plasma CETP levels in *CETP* 405V homozygotes [250], is associated with longevity. However, the direction and the magnitude of this effect is not clear as some studies have found a positive association, some a negative association, and some no association with longevity [251-256]. It has also been shown that in young adults, this allele is associated with higher fractional anisotropy, a measure of myelination in brain's white matter [257]. In older subjects, however, this effect is reversed [257]. Furthermore, genetic studies have proposed a relationship between C629A, I405V, and D442G *CETP* polymorphisms and AD risk. Intriguingly, the effects that are exerted by these polymorphisms may be dependent on the presence of the *APOE4* allele. Rodriguez et al. reported that in *APOE4* carriers, the AA genotype of the C629A *CETP* polymorphism is associated with lower AD risk [258]. It has also been shown that in the Northern Han Chinese population, there is an association between the G allele of the D442G *CETP* polymorphism and lower AD risk, an effect that was abolished in the absence of *APOE4* [259]. Additionally, Murphy et al. reported that in *APOE4* non-carriers, the I allele of the I405V polymorphism is protective, whereas the V allele is associated with higher AD risk [260]. Interestingly, these associations are reversed in *APOE4* carriers [260]. These results are replicated by the Rotterdam study [250]. However, the Einstein Aging Study reported an association between the VV genotype and slower memory decline and AD risk, and a recent meta-analysis by Li et al. reported no association between AD and the 1405V *CETP* polymorphism [253, 261]. Clearly, more research is required to elucidate the specific role of CETP in the brain and its contribution to AD.

3.5. ApoE receptors

APP endocytosis is regulated by several members of the lipoprotein receptor family leading to increased or reduced Aβ generation [74]. These receptors are also critical for Aβ clearance. LRP1 can bind Aβ directly or bind apoE-associated Aβ to internalize and transport soluble Aβ across the BBB to plasma for eventual degradation, or mediate degradation within cell lysosomes [262-266]. *APOE* genotype impacts clearance of Aβ-apoE complexes with Aβ-apoE4 having the slowest net clearance rate [267]. Findings in knockout mice imply LDLR may also enhance Aβ clearance [268, 269]. Other apolipoproteins such as clusterin may play a role in mediating Aβ degradation and clearance though the LDLR family of receptors [83]. In addition to Aβ removal, apoE receptors also regulate tau phosphorylation. Reelin signaling through apoER2 and VLDLR inhibits the activity of GSK- 3β and blockade of this pathway increases hyperphosphorylated tau in the brain [270, 271]. Although apoE receptors are clearly implicated in AD pathogenesis by a number of mechanisms, genetic evidence for their role is not robust, despite mutations in *LDLR* being highly associated with hypercholesterolemia in humans [272]. For example, a polymorphism in exon 3 of the *LRP1* gene (rs1799986) has been weakly correlated with increased risk of AD, although subjects with both this *LRP1* allele and a tau polymorphism (*MAPT*, intron 9, rs2471738) have 6.2-fold higher risk of developing AD than those without this genotype [273-275]. A polymorphism in *LRP2* (rs3755166) has also been reported to be associated with AD [276, 277]. By contrast, the neuronal sortilin-related receptor (*SORL1*, also known as *LR11*) is an apoE receptor that has been shown to be significantly associated with AD risk by multiple groups and in a GWAS [278, 279]. SORL1 levels are reduced in AD brains [280] and risk variants that decrease SORL1 expression, particularly in childhood and adolescence, predict increases in amyloid pathology [281].

4. Conclusions and future directions

ApoE is the major apolipoprotein produced within the CNS and is intimately involved in the risk, progression, and pathogenesis of AD. Allelic differences in *APOE* appear to confer isoform specific effects with respect to Aβ deposition, degradation and clearance, tau phosphorylation, neuronal injury and inflammation. Given its gain of toxic or loss of beneficial function, strategies aimed at increasing functional apoE may be of therapeutic interest, although it is possible that elevated levels of dysfunctional apoE4 may actually be detrimental for *APOE4* carriers. However, as over 50% of AD patients carry at least one *APOE4* allele, development of future therapies must take into account the structural and functional differences of this lipoprotein isoform, and seek to develop ways to either correct or bypass the "dysfunction" of apoE4. Long ignored, the importance of clusterin in CNS health and disease is now rapidly expanding. While clinical evidence is mounting that clusterin may be involved in AD disease risk, severity, and rate of decline both with respect to cognitive function and Aβ metabolism, the mechanism(s) by which clusterin confers these roles is poorly understood. ApoA-I may also influence AD pathology, potentially by modulating cerebrovascular integrity and function by assisting in the removal of Aβ peptides from cerebrovascular smooth muscle cells and decreasing inflammation. Indeed, the known effects of common AD comorbidities such as type II diabetes and hypercholesterolemia, on apoA-I function, should be taken into account in clinical studies on dementia risk and potential therapeutic approaches.

In the cardiovascular field, many preclinical and clinical studies have endeavored to increase the net concentration of circulating HDL to protect against cardiovascular disease. Many of these studies may also have implications for CNS function. However, as some of these approaches, such as the inhibition of CETP, have failed to meet their primary endpoints for cardiovascular disease despite significantly increasing HDL cholesterol levels, the lipoprotein field is now deeply invested in understanding the functional complexities of HDL. Therapeutic interventions aimed at increasing the function of HDL particles and their cargo may be of much greater importance than increasing its net levels, in both the peripheral and CNS compartments. Given the complexity of the HDL proteome and lipidome, it will be critical to divest the same details in the CNS to allow for therapeutic development targeting lipoprotein species.

Author details

Sophie Stukas, Iva Kulic, Shahab Zareyan and Cheryl L. Wellington*

*Address all correspondence to: wcheryl@mail.ubc.ca

Department of Pathology and Laboratory Medicine, Djavad Mowafaghian Centre for Brain Health, University of British Columbia, Vancouver, British Columbia, Canada

References

[1] Dietschy JM. Central nervous system: cholesterol turnover, brain development and neurodegeneration. Biological chemistry. 2009 Apr;390(4):287-93.

[2] Lim L, Wenk MR. Neuronal Membrane Lipids – Their Role in the Synaptic Vesicle Cycle. In: Tettamanti GG, G., editor. Handbook of Neurochemistry and Molecular Neurobiology. New York: Springer Science+Business Media; 2009. p. 223 - 38.

[3] Vance JE, Hayashi H. Formation and function of apolipoprotein E-containing lipoproteins in the nervous system. Biochimica et biophysica acta. 2010 Aug;1801(8): 806-18.

[4] Beffert U, Danik M, Krzywkowski P, Ramassamy C, Berrada F, Poirier J. The neurobiology of apolipoproteins and their receptors in the CNS and Alzheimer's disease. Brain research Brain research reviews. 1998 Jul;27(2):119-42.

[5] Pitas RE, Boyles JK, Lee SH, Hui D, Weisgraber KH. Lipoproteins and their receptors in the central nervous system. Characterization of the lipoproteins in cerebrospinal fluid and identification of apolipoprotein B,E(LDL) receptors in the brain. The Journal of biological chemistry. 1987 Oct 15;262(29):14352-60.

[6] Ladu MJ, Reardon C, Van Eldik L, Fagan AM, Bu G, Holtzman D, et al. Lipoproteins in the central nervous system. Annals of the New York Academy of Sciences. 2000 Apr;903:167-75.

[7] LaDu MJ, Gilligan SM, Lukens JR, Cabana VG, Reardon CA, Van Eldik LJ, et al. Nascent astrocyte particles differ from lipoproteins in CSF. Journal of neurochemistry. 1998 May;70(5):2070-81.

[8] Koch S, Donarski N, Goetze K, Kreckel M, Stuerenburg HJ, Buhmann C, et al. Characterization of four lipoprotein classes in human cerebrospinal fluid. Journal of lipid research. 2001 Jul;42(7):1143-51.

[9] Borghini I, Barja F, Pometta D, James RW. Characterization of subpopulations of lipoprotein particles isolated from human cerebrospinal fluid. Biochimica et biophysica acta. 1995 Mar 16;1255(2):192-200.

[10] DeMattos RB, Brendza RP, Heuser JE, Kierson M, Cirrito JR, Fryer J, et al. Purification and characterization of astrocyte-secreted apolipoprotein E and J-containing lipoproteins from wild-type and human apoE transgenic mice. Neurochemistry international. 2001 Nov- Dec;39(5-6):415-25.

[11] Roheim PS, Carey M, Forte T, Vega GL. Apolipoproteins in human cerebrospinal fluid. Proceedings of the National Academy of Sciences of the United States of America. 1979 Sep;76(9):4646-9.

[12] Fan J, Shimizu Y, Chan J, Wilkinson A, Ito A, Tontonoz P, et al. Hormonal modulators of glial ABCA1 and apoE levels. Journal of lipid research. 2013 Nov;54(11): 3139-50.

[13] Demeester N, Castro G, Desrumaux C, De Geitere C, Fruchart JC, Santens P, et al. Characterization and functional studies of lipoproteins, lipid transfer proteins, and lecithin:cholesterol acyltransferase in CSF of normal individuals and patients with Alzheimer's disease. Journal of lipid research. 2000 Jun;41(6):963-74.

[14] Stukas S, Robert J, Wellington CL. High Density Lipoproteins and Cerebrovasular Integrity in Alzheimer's Disease. Cell metabolism. 2014.

[15] Roher AE, Maarouf CL, Sue LI, Hu Y, Wilson J, Beach TG. Proteomics-derived cerebrospinal fluid markers of autopsy-confirmed Alzheimer's disease. Biomarkers : biochemical indicators of exposure, response, and susceptibility to chemicals. 2009 Nov; 14(7):493-501.

[16] Wahrle SE, Shah AR, Fagan AM, Smemo S, Kauwe JS, Grupe A, et al. Apolipoprotein E levels in cerebrospinal fluid and the effects of ABCA1 polymorphisms. Molecular neurodegeneration. 2007;2:7.

[17] Ulrich JD, Burchett JM, Restivo JL, Schuler DR, Verghese PB, Mahan TE, et al. In vivo measurement of apolipoprotein E from the brain interstitial fluid using microdialysis. Molecular neurodegeneration. 2013;8:13.

[18] Fagan AM, Holtzman DM, Munson G, Mathur T, Schneider D, Chang LK, et al. Unique lipoproteins secreted by primary astrocytes from wild type, apoE (-/-), and human apoE transgenic mice. The Journal of biological chemistry. 1999 Oct 15;274(42):30001-7.

[19] Dorey E, Chang N, Liu QY, Yang Z, Zhang W. Apolipoprotein E, amyloid-beta, and neuroinflammation in Alzheimer's disease. Neuroscience bulletin. 2014 Apr;30(2): 317-30.

[20] Hirsch-Reinshagen V, Zhou S, Burgess BL, Bernier L, McIsaac SA, Chan JY, et al. Deficiency of ABCA1 impairs apolipoprotein E metabolism in brain. The Journal of biological chemistry. 2004 Sep 24;279(39):41197-207.

[21] Wahrle SE, Jiang H, Parsadanian M, Legleiter J, Han X, Fryer JD, et al. ABCA1 is required for normal central nervous system ApoE levels and for lipidation of astrocyte-secreted apoE. The Journal of biological chemistry. 2004 Sep 24;279(39):40987-93.

[22] Hatters DM, Peters-Libeu CA, Weisgraber KH. Apolipoprotein E structure: insights into function. Trends in biochemical sciences. 2006 Aug;31(8):445-54.

[23] Liu CC, Kanekiyo T, Xu H, Bu G. Apolipoprotein E and Alzheimer disease: risk, mechanisms and therapy. Nature reviews Neurology. 2013 Feb;9(2):106-18.

[24] de Silva HV, Harmony JA, Stuart WD, Gil CM, Robbins J. Apolipoprotein J: structure and tissue distribution. Biochemistry. 1990 Jun 5;29(22):5380-9.

[25] Lidstrom AM, Hesse C, Rosengren L, Fredman P, Davidsson P, Blennow K. Normal levels of clusterin in cerebrospinal fluid in Alzheimer's disease, and no change after acute ischemic stroke. Journal of Alzheimer's disease : JAD. 2001 Oct;3(5):435-42.

[26] Rizzi F, Coletta M, Bettuzzi S. Chapter 2: Clusterin (CLU): From one gene and two transcripts to many proteins. Advances in cancer research. 2009;104:9-23.

[27] Yu JT, Tan L. The role of clusterin in Alzheimer's disease: pathways, pathogenesis, and therapy. Molecular neurobiology. 2012 Apr;45(2):314-26.

[28] Elshourbagy NA, Boguski MS, Liao WS, Jefferson LS, Gordon JI, Taylor JM. Expression of rat apolipoprotein A-IV and A-I genes: mRNA induction during development and in response to glucocorticoids and insulin. Proceedings of the National Academy of Sciences of the United States of America. 1985 Dec;82(23):8242-6.

[29] Zannis VI, Cole FS, Jackson CL, Kurnit DM, Karathanasis SK. Distribution of apolipoprotein A-I, C-II, C-III, and E mRNA in fetal human tissues. Time-dependent induction of apolipoprotein E mRNA by cultures of human monocyte-macrophages. Biochemistry. 1985 Jul 30;24(16):4450-5.

[30] Karasinska JM, Rinninger F, Lutjohann D, Ruddle P, Franciosi S, Kruit JK, et al. Specific loss of brain ABCA1 increases brain cholesterol uptake and influences neuronal structure and function. The Journal of neuroscience : the official journal of the Society for Neuroscience. 2009 Mar 18;29(11):3579-89.

[31] Stukas S, Robert J, Lee M, Kulic I, Carr M, Tourigny K, et al. Intravenously injected human apolipoprotein A-I rapidly enters the central nervous system via the choroid plexus. Journal of the American Heart Association. Forthcoming 2014.

[32] Kratzer I, Wernig K, Panzenboeck U, Bernhart E, Reicher H, Wronski R, et al. Apolipoprotein A-I coating of protamine-oligonucleotide nanoparticles increases particle uptake and transcytosis in an in vitro model of the blood-brain barrier. Journal of controlled release : official journal of the Controlled Release Society. 2007 Feb 26;117(3):301-11.

[33] Song H, Seishima M, Saito K, Maeda S, Takemura M, Noma A, et al. Apo A-I and apo E concentrations in cerebrospinal fluids of patients with acute meningitis. Annals of clinical biochemistry. 1998 May;35 (Pt 3):408-14.

[34] Navarro A, Tolivia J, Astudillo A, del Valle E. Pattern of apolipoprotein D immunoreactivity in human brain. Neuroscience letters. 1998 Sep 18;254(1):17-20.

[35] Dassati S, Waldner A, Schweigreiter R. Apolipoprotein D takes center stage in the stress response of the aging and degenerative brain. Neurobiology of aging. 2014 Jul;35(7):1632-42.

[36] Koldamova RP, Lefterov IM, Ikonomovic MD, Skoko J, Lefterov PI, Isanski BA, et al. 22R-hydroxycholesterol and 9-cis-retinoic acid induce ATP-binding cassette transporter A1 expression and cholesterol efflux in brain cells and decrease amyloid beta secretion. The Journal of biological chemistry. 2003 Apr 11;278(15):13244-56.

[37] Kim WS, Rahmanto AS, Kamili A, Rye KA, Guillemin GJ, Gelissen IC, et al. Role of ABCG1 and ABCA1 in regulation of neuronal cholesterol efflux to apolipoprotein E discs and suppression of amyloid-beta peptide generation. The Journal of biological chemistry. 2007 Feb 2;282(5):2851-61.

[38] Panzenboeck U, Balazs Z, Sovic A, Hrzenjak A, Levak-Frank S, Wintersperger A, et al. ABCA1 and scavenger receptor class B, type I, are modulators of reverse sterol transport at an in vitro blood-brain barrier constituted of porcine brain capillary endothelial cells. The Journal of biological chemistry. 2002 Nov 8;277(45):42781-9.

[39] Saint-Pol J, Vandenhaute E, Boucau MC, Candela P, Dehouck L, Cecchelli R, et al. Brain pericytes ABCA1 expression mediates cholesterol efflux but not cellular amyloid-beta peptide accumulation. Journal of Alzheimer's disease : JAD. 2012;30(3):489-503.

[40] Stukas S, May S, Wilkinson A, Chan J, Donkin J, Wellington CL. The LXR agonist GW3965 increases apoA-I protein levels in the central nervous system independent of ABCA1. Biochimica et biophysica acta. 2012 Mar;1821(3):536-46.

[41] Kim WS, Guillemin GJ, Glaros EN, Lim CK, Garner B. Quantitation of ATP-binding cassette subfamily-A transporter gene expression in primary human brain cells. Neuroreport. 2006 Jun 26;17(9):891-6.

[42] Wang N, Lan D, Gerbod-Giannone M, Linsel-Nitschke P, Jehle AW, Chen W, et al. ATP-binding cassette transporter A7 (ABCA7) binds apolipoprotein A-I and mediates cellular phospholipid but not cholesterol efflux. The Journal of biological chemistry. 2003 Oct 31;278(44):42906-12.

[43] Kim WS, Fitzgerald ML, Kang K, Okuhira K, Bell SA, Manning JJ, et al. Abca7 null mice retain normal macrophage phosphatidylcholine and cholesterol efflux activity despite alterations in adipose mass and serum cholesterol levels. The Journal of biological chemistry. 2005 Feb 4;280(5):3989-95.

[44] Iwamoto N, Abe-Dohmae S, Sato R, Yokoyama S. ABCA7 expression is regulated by cellular cholesterol through the SREBP2 pathway and associated with phagocytosis. Journal of lipid research. 2006 Sep;47(9):1915-27.

[45] Tanaka N, Abe-Dohmae S, Iwamoto N, Fitzgerald ML, Yokoyama S. Helical apolipoproteins of high-density lipoprotein enhance phagocytosis by stabilizing ATP-binding cassette transporter A7. Journal of lipid research. 2010 Sep;51(9):2591-9.

[46] Wang N, Lan D, Chen W, Matsuura F, Tall AR. ATP-binding cassette transporters G1 and G4 mediate cellular cholesterol efflux to high-density lipoproteins. Proceedings of the National Academy of Sciences of the United States of America. 2004 Jun 29;101(26):9774- 9.

[47] Tarr PT, Edwards PA. ABCG1 and ABCG4 are coexpressed in neurons and astrocytes of the CNS and regulate cholesterol homeostasis through SREBP-2. Journal of lipid research. 2008 Jan;49(1):169-82.

[48] Wang N, Yvan-Charvet L, Lutjohann D, Mulder M, Vanmierlo T, Kim TW, et al. ATP- binding cassette transporters G1 and G4 mediate cholesterol and desmosterol efflux to HDL and regulate sterol accumulation in the brain. FASEB journal : official publication of the Federation of American Societies for Experimental Biology. 2008 Apr;22(4):1073-82.

[49] Albers JJ, Marcovina SM, Christenson RH. Lecithin cholesterol acyltransferase in human cerebrospinal fluid: reduced level in patients with multiple sclerosis and evidence of direct synthesis in the brain. International journal of clinical & laboratory research. 1992;22(3):169-72.

[50] Warden CH, Langner CA, Gordon JI, Taylor BA, McLean JW, Lusis AJ. Tissue-specific expression, developmental regulation, and chromosomal mapping of the lecithin: cholesterol acyltransferase gene. Evidence for expression in brain and testes as well as liver. The Journal of biological chemistry. 1989 Dec 25;264(36):21573-81.

[51] Yamada T, Kawata M, Arai H, Fukasawa M, Inoue K, Sato T. Astroglial localization of cholesteryl ester transfer protein in normal and Alzheimer's disease brain tissues. Acta neuropathologica. 1995;90(6):633-6.

[52] Lagrost L, Athias A, Gambert P, Lallemant C. Comparative study of phospholipid transfer activities mediated by cholesteryl ester transfer protein and phospholipid transfer protein. Journal of lipid research. 1994 May;35(5):825-35.

[53] Albers JJ, Vuletic S, Cheung MC. Role of plasma phospholipid transfer protein in lipid and lipoprotein metabolism. Biochimica et biophysica acta. 2012 Mar;1821(3): 345-57.

[54] Calabresi L, Simonelli S, Gomaraschi M, Franceschini G. Genetic lecithin:cholesterol acyltransferase deficiency and cardiovascular disease. Atherosclerosis. 2012 Jun; 222(2):299-306.

[55] Hirsch-Reinshagen V, Donkin J, Stukas S, Chan J, Wilkinson A, Fan J, et al. LCAT synthesized by primary astrocytes esterifies cholesterol on glia-derived lipoproteins. Journal of lipid research. 2009 May;50(5):885-93.

[56] Guyton JR, Miller SE, Martin ME, Khan WA, Roses AD, Strittmatter WJ. Novel large apolipoprotein E-containing lipoproteins of density 1.006-1.060 g/ml in human cerebrospinal fluid. Journal of neurochemistry. 1998 Mar;70(3):1235-40.

[57] Albers JJ, Wolfbauer G, Cheung MC, Day JR, Ching AF, Lok S, et al. Functional expression of human and mouse plasma phospholipid transfer protein: effect of recombinant and plasma PLTP on HDL subspecies. Biochimica et biophysica acta. 1995 Aug 24;1258(1):27-34.

[58] Chirackal Manavalan AP, Kober A, Metso J, Lang I, Becker T, Hasslitzer K, et al. Phospholipid transfer protein is expressed in cerebrovascular endothelial cells and involved in high density lipoprotein biogenesis and remodeling at the blood-brain barrier. The Journal of biological chemistry. 2014 Feb 21;289(8):4683-98.

[59] Gander R, Eller P, Kaser S, Theurl I, Walter D, Sauper T, et al. Molecular characterization of rabbit phospholipid transfer protein: choroid plexus and ependyma synthesize high levels of phospholipid transfer protein. Journal of lipid research. 2002 Apr; 43(4):636-45.

[60] Oslakovic C, Krisinger MJ, Andersson A, Jauhiainen M, Ehnholm C, Dahlback B. Anionic phospholipids lose their procoagulant properties when incorporated into high density lipoproteins. The Journal of biological chemistry. 2009 Feb 27;284(9): 5896-904.

[61] Zhou T, He Q, Tong Y, Zhan R, Xu F, Fan D, et al. Phospholipid transfer protein (PLTP) deficiency impaired blood-brain barrier integrity by increasing cerebrovascular oxidative stress. Biochemical and biophysical research communications. 2014 Mar 7;445(2):352-6.

[62] Vuletic S, Jin LW, Marcovina SM, Peskind ER, Moller T, Albers JJ. Widespread distribution of PLTP in human CNS: evidence for PLTP synthesis by glia and neurons, and increased levels in Alzheimer's disease. Journal of lipid research. 2003 Jun;44(6): 1113-23.

[63] Vuletic S, Peskind ER, Marcovina SM, Quinn JF, Cheung MC, Kennedy H, et al. Reduced CSF PLTP activity in Alzheimer's disease and other neurologic diseases; PLTP induces ApoE secretion in primary human astrocytes in vitro. Journal of neuroscience research. 2005 May 1;80(3):406-13.

[64] Dong W, Albers JJ, Vuletic S. Phospholipid transfer protein reduces phosphorylation of tau in human neuronal cells. Journal of neuroscience research. 2009 Nov 1;87(14): 3176-85.

[65] Kingwell BA, Chapman MJ, Kontush A, Miller NE. HDL-targeted therapies: progress, failures and future. Nature reviews Drug discovery. 2014 Jun;13(6):445-64.

[66] Albers JJ, Tollefson JH, Wolfbauer G, Albright RE, Jr. Cholesteryl ester transfer protein in human brain. International journal of clinical & laboratory research. 1992;21(3):264-6.

[67] Pape ME, Rehberg EF, Marotti KR, Melchior GW. Molecular cloning, sequence, and expression of cynomolgus monkey cholesteryl ester transfer protein. Inverse correlation between hepatic cholesteryl ester transfer protein mRNA levels and plasma high density lipoprotein levels. Arteriosclerosis and thrombosis : a journal of vascular biology / American Heart Association. 1991 Nov-Dec;11(6):1759-71.

[68] Bu G. Apolipoprotein E and its receptors in Alzheimer's disease: pathways, pathogenesis and therapy. Nature reviews Neuroscience. 2009 May;10(5):333-44.

[69] Holtzman DM, Herz J, Bu G. Apolipoprotein E and apolipoprotein E receptors: normal biology and roles in Alzheimer disease. Cold Spring Harbor perspectives in medicine. 2012 Mar;2(3):a006312.

[70] Fryer JD, Demattos RB, McCormick LM, O'Dell MA, Spinner ML, Bales KR, et al. The low density lipoprotein receptor regulates the level of central nervous system human and murine apolipoprotein E but does not modify amyloid plaque pathology in PDAPP mice. The Journal of biological chemistry. 2005 Jul 8;280(27):25754-9.

[71] Kim J, Castellano JM, Jiang H, Basak JM, Parsadanian M, Pham V, et al. Overexpression of low-density lipoprotein receptor in the brain markedly inhibits amyloid deposition and increases extracellular A beta clearance. Neuron. 2009 Dec 10;64(5):632-44.

[72] Liu Q, Zerbinatti CV, Zhang J, Hoe HS, Wang B, Cole SL, et al. Amyloid precursor protein regulates brain apolipoprotein E and cholesterol metabolism through lipoprotein receptor LRP1. Neuron. 2007 Oct 4;56(1):66-78.

[73] Zerbinatti CV, Wahrle SE, Kim H, Cam JA, Bales K, Paul SM, et al. Apolipoprotein E and low density lipoprotein receptor-related protein facilitate intraneuronal Abeta42 accumulation in amyloid model mice. The Journal of biological chemistry. 2006 Nov 24;281(47):36180-6.

[74] Lane-Donovan C, Philips GT, Herz J. More than Cholesterol Transporters: Lipoprotein Receptors in CNS Function and Neurodegeneration. Neuron. 2014 Aug 20;83(4):771-87.

[75] Rice DS, Curran T. Role of the reelin signaling pathway in central nervous system development. Annual review of neuroscience. 2001;24:1005-39.

[76] Herz J, Chen Y. Reelin, lipoprotein receptors and synaptic plasticity. Nature reviews Neuroscience. 2006 Nov;7(11):850-9.

[77] Leeb C, Eresheim C, Nimpf J. Clusterin is a ligand for apolipoprotein E receptor 2 (ApoER2) and very low density lipoprotein receptor (VLDLR) and signals via the Reelin- signaling pathway. The Journal of biological chemistry. 2014 Feb 14;289(7): 4161-72.

[78] Christie RH, Chung H, Rebeck GW, Strickland D, Hyman BT. Expression of the very low-density lipoprotein receptor (VLDL-r), an apolipoprotein-E receptor, in the central nervous system and in Alzheimer's disease. Journal of neuropathology and experimental neurology. 1996 Apr;55(4):491-8.

[79] Clatworthy AE, Stockinger W, Christie RH, Schneider WJ, Nimpf J, Hyman BT, et al. Expression and alternate splicing of apolipoprotein E receptor 2 in brain. Neuroscience. 1999 Mar;90(3):903-11.

[80] Moestrup SK, Gliemann J, Pallesen G. Distribution of the alpha 2-macroglobulin receptor/low density lipoprotein receptor-related protein in human tissues. Cell and tissue research. 1992 Sep;269(3):375-82.

[81] Rapp A, Gmeiner B, Huttinger M. Implication of apoE isoforms in cholesterol metabolism by primary rat hippocampal neurons and astrocytes. Biochimie. 2006 May; 88(5):473-83.

[82] Rebeck GW, LaDu MJ, Estus S, Bu G, Weeber EJ. The generation and function of soluble apoE receptors in the CNS. Molecular neurodegeneration. 2006;1:15.

[83] Spuch C, Ortolano S, Navarro C. LRP-1 and LRP-2 receptors function in the membrane neuron. Trafficking mechanisms and proteolytic processing in Alzheimer's disease. Frontiers in physiology. 2012;3:269.

[84] Motoi Y, Aizawa T, Haga S, Nakamura S, Namba Y, Ikeda K. Neuronal localization of a novel mosaic apolipoprotein E receptor, LR11, in rat and human brain. Brain research. 1999 Jul 3;833(2):209-15.

[85] Hyman BT, Phelps CH, Beach TG, Bigio EH, Cairns NJ, Carrillo MC, et al. National Institute on Aging-Alzheimer's Association guidelines for the neuropathologic assessment of Alzheimer's disease. Alzheimer's & dementia : the journal of the Alzheimer's Association. 2012 Jan;8(1):1-13.

[86] Zlokovic BV. Neurovascular pathways to neurodegeneration in Alzheimer's disease and other disorders. Nature reviews Neuroscience. 2011 Dec;12(12):723-38.

[87] de la Torre JC. Alzheimer disease as a vascular disorder: nosological evidence. Stroke; a journal of cerebral circulation. 2002 Apr;33(4):1152-62.

[88] Gorelick PB. Risk factors for vascular dementia and Alzheimer disease. Stroke; a journal of cerebral circulation. 2004 Nov;35(11 Suppl 1):2620-2.

[89] Hayden KM, Zandi PP, Lyketsos CG, Khachaturian AS, Bastian LA, Charoonruk G, et al. Vascular risk factors for incident Alzheimer disease and vascular dementia: the

Cache County study. Alzheimer disease and associated disorders. 2006 Apr-Jun; 20(2):93-100.

[90] Kalaria RN. The role of cerebral ischemia in Alzheimer's disease. Neurobiology of aging. 2000 Mar-Apr;21(2):321-30.

[91] Esiri MM, Nagy Z, Smith MZ, Barnetson L, Smith AD. Cerebrovascular disease and threshold for dementia in the early stages of Alzheimer's disease. Lancet. 1999 Sep 11;354(9182):919-20.

[92] Petrovitch H, Ross GW, Steinhorn SC, Abbott RD, Markesbery W, Davis D, et al. AD lesions and infarcts in demented and non-demented Japanese-American men. Annals of neurology. 2005 Jan;57(1):98-103.

[93] Snowdon DA, Greiner LH, Mortimer JA, Riley KP, Greiner PA, Markesbery WR. Brain infarction and the clinical expression of Alzheimer disease. The Nun Study. Jama. 1997 Mar 12;277(10):813-7.

[94] Honjo K, van Reekum R, Verhoeff NP. Alzheimer's disease and infection: do infectious agents contribute to progression of Alzheimer's disease? Alzheimer's & dementia : the journal of the Alzheimer's Association. 2009 Jul;5(4):348-60.

[95] Kalaria RN, Bhatti SU, Lust WD, Perry G. The amyloid precursor protein in ischemic brain injury and chronic hypoperfusion. Annals of the New York Academy of Sciences. 1993 Sep 24;695:190-3.

[96] Nihashi T, Inao S, Kajita Y, Kawai T, Sugimoto T, Niwa M, et al. Expression and distribution of beta amyloid precursor protein and beta amyloid peptide in reactive astrocytes after transient middle cerebral artery occlusion. Acta neurochirurgica. 2001;143(3):287-95.

[97] Takeda S, Sato N, Morishita R. Systemic inflammation, blood-brain barrier vulnerability and cognitive/non-cognitive symptoms in Alzheimer disease: relevance to pathogenesis and therapy. Frontiers in aging neuroscience. 2014;6:171.

[98] Foley P. Lipids in Alzheimer's disease: A century-old story. Biochimica et biophysica acta. 2010 Aug;1801(8):750-3.

[99] Di Paolo G, Kim TW. Linking lipids to Alzheimer's disease: cholesterol and beyond. Nature reviews Neuroscience. 2011 May;12(5):284-96.

[100] Kosicek M, Hecimovic S. Phospholipids and Alzheimer's disease: alterations, mechanisms and potential biomarkers. International journal of molecular sciences. 2013;14(1):1310-22.

[101] Han X, Fagan AM, Cheng H, Morris JC, Xiong C, Holtzman DM. Cerebrospinal fluid sulfatide is decreased in subjects with incipient dementia. Annals of neurology. 2003 Jul;54(1):115-9.

[102] Satoi H, Tomimoto H, Ohtani R, Kitano T, Kondo T, Watanabe M, et al. Astroglial expression of ceramide in Alzheimer's disease brains: a role during neuronal apoptosis. Neuroscience. 2005;130(3):657-66.

[103] Soderberg M, Edlund C, Kristensson K, Dallner G. Fatty acid composition of brain phospholipids in aging and in Alzheimer's disease. Lipids. 1991 Jun;26(6):421-5.

[104] Tully AM, Roche HM, Doyle R, Fallon C, Bruce I, Lawlor B, et al. Low serum cholesteryl ester-docosahexaenoic acid levels in Alzheimer's disease: a case-control study. The British journal of nutrition. 2003 Apr;89(4):483-9.

[105] Bennett SA, Valenzuela N, Xu H, Franko B, Fai S, Figeys D. Using neurolipidomics to identify phospholipid mediators of synaptic (dys)function in Alzheimer's Disease. Frontiers in physiology. 2013;4:168.

[106] Estus S, Golde TE, Younkin SG. Normal processing of the Alzheimer's disease amyloid beta protein precursor generates potentially amyloidogenic carboxyl-terminal derivatives. Annals of the New York Academy of Sciences. 1992 Dec 31;674:138-48.

[107] Haass C, Selkoe DJ. Cellular processing of beta-amyloid precursor protein and the genesis of amyloid beta-peptide. Cell. 1993 Dec 17;75(6):1039-42.

[108] Seubert P, Vigo-Pelfrey C, Esch F, Lee M, Dovey H, Davis D, et al. Isolation and quantification of soluble Alzheimer's beta-peptide from biological fluids. Nature. 1992 Sep 24;359(6393):325-7.

[109] Masters CL, Selkoe DJ. Biochemistry of amyloid beta-protein and amyloid deposits in Alzheimer disease. Cold Spring Harbor perspectives in medicine. 2012 Jun; 2(6):a006262.

[110] Haass C, Kaether C, Thinakaran G, Sisodia S. Trafficking and proteolytic processing of APP. Cold Spring Harbor perspectives in medicine. 2012 May;2(5):a006270.

[111] Grziwa B, Grimm MO, Masters CL, Beyreuther K, Hartmann T, Lichtenthaler SF. The transmembrane domain of the amyloid precursor protein in microsomal membranes is on both sides shorter than predicted. The Journal of biological chemistry. 2003 Feb 28;278(9):6803-8.

[112] Vetrivel KS, Thinakaran G. Membrane rafts in Alzheimer's disease beta-amyloid production. Biochimica et biophysica acta. 2010 Aug;1801(8):860-7.

[113] Grimm MO, Grimm HS, Patzold AJ, Zinser EG, Halonen R, Duering M, et al. Regulation of cholesterol and sphingomyelin metabolism by amyloid-beta and presenilin. Nature cell biology. 2005 Nov;7(11):1118-23.

[114] Sawamura N, Ko M, Yu W, Zou K, Hanada K, Suzuki T, et al. Modulation of amyloid precursor protein cleavage by cellular sphingolipids. The Journal of biological chemistry. 2004 Mar 19;279(12):11984-91.

[115] Puglielli L, Ellis BC, Saunders AJ, Kovacs DM. Ceramide stabilizes beta-site amyloid precursor protein-cleaving enzyme 1 and promotes amyloid beta-peptide biogenesis. The Journal of biological chemistry. 2003 May 30;278(22):19777-83.

[116] Haass C, Schlossmacher MG, Hung AY, Vigo-Pelfrey C, Mellon A, Ostaszewski BL, et al. Amyloid beta-peptide is produced by cultured cells during normal metabolism. Nature. 1992 Sep 24;359(6393):322-5.

[117] Shoji M, Golde TE, Ghiso J, Cheung TT, Estus S, Shaffer LM, et al. Production of the Alzheimer amyloid beta protein by normal proteolytic processing. Science. 1992 Oct 2;258(5079):126-9.

[118] Tanzi RE. The genetics of Alzheimer disease. Cold Spring Harbor perspectives in medicine. 2012 Oct;2(10).

[119] Mawuenyega KG, Sigurdson W, Ovod V, Munsell L, Kasten T, Morris JC, et al. De-creased clearance of CNS beta-amyloid in Alzheimer's disease. Science. 2010 Dec 24;330(6012):1774.

[120] Kanekiyo T, Xu H, Bu G. ApoE and Abeta in Alzheimer's disease: accidental encoun-ters or partners? Neuron. 2014 Feb 19;81(4):740-54.

[121] Tanzi RE, Moir RD, Wagner SL. Clearance of Alzheimer's Abeta peptide: the many roads to perdition. Neuron. 2004 Sep 2;43(5):605-8.

[122] Wildsmith KR, Holley M, Savage JC, Skerrett R, Landreth GE. Evidence for impaired amyloid beta clearance in Alzheimer's disease. Alzheimer's research & therapy. 2013;5(4):33.

[123] Corder EH, Saunders AM, Strittmatter WJ, Schmechel DE, Gaskell PC, Small GW, et al. Gene dose of apolipoprotein E type 4 allele and the risk of Alzheimer's disease in late onset families. Science. 1993 Aug 13;261(5123):921-3.

[124] Farrer LA, Cupples LA, Haines JL, Hyman B, Kukull WA, Mayeux R, et al. Effects of age, sex, and ethnicity on the association between apolipoprotein E genotype and Alzheimer disease. A meta-analysis. APOE and Alzheimer Disease Meta Analysis Consortium. Jama. 1997 Oct 22-29;278(16):1349-56.

[125] Ward A, Crean S, Mercaldi CJ, Collins JM, Boyd D, Cook MN, et al. Prevalence of apolipoprotein E4 genotype and homozygotes (APOE e4/4) among patients diag-nosed with Alzheimer's disease: a systematic review and meta-analysis. Neuroepi-demiology. 2012;38(1):1-17.

[126] Rebeck GW, Reiter JS, Strickland DK, Hyman BT. Apolipoprotein E in sporadic Alz-heimer's disease: allelic variation and receptor interactions. Neuron. 1993 Oct;11(4): 575- 80.

[127] Strittmatter WJ, Saunders AM, Schmechel D, Pericak-Vance M, Enghild J, Salvesen GS, et al. Apolipoprotein E: high-avidity binding to beta-amyloid and increased fre-quency of type 4 allele in late-onset familial Alzheimer disease. Proceedings of the

National Academy of Sciences of the United States of America. 1993 Mar 1;90(5): 1977-81.

[128] Verghese PB, Castellano JM, Holtzman DM. Apolipoprotein E in Alzheimer's disease and other neurological disorders. Lancet neurology. 2011 Mar;10(3):241-52.

[129] Garai K, Verghese PB, Baban B, Holtzman DM, Frieden C. The Binding of Apolipo-protein E to Oligomers and Fibrils of Amyloid-beta Alters the Kinetics of Amyloid Aggregation. Biochemistry. 2014 Sep 25.

[130] Zlokovic BV. Cerebrovascular effects of apolipoprotein E: implications for Alzheimer disease. JAMA neurology. 2013 Apr;70(4):440-4.

[131] Chalmers K, Wilcock GK, Love S. APOE epsilon 4 influences the pathological pheno-type of Alzheimer's disease by favouring cerebrovascular over parenchymal accumu-lation of A beta protein. Neuropathology and applied neurobiology. 2003 Jun;29(3): 231-8.

[132] Premkumar DR, Cohen DL, Hedera P, Friedland RP, Kalaria RN. Apolipoprotein E-epsilon4 alleles in cerebral amyloid angiopathy and cerebrovascular pathology asso-ciated with Alzheimer's disease. The American journal of pathology. 1996 Jun;148(6): 2083-95.

[133] Mak AC, Pullinger CR, Tang LF, Wong JS, Deo RC, Schwarz JM, et al. Effects of the Absence of Apolipoprotein E on Lipoproteins, Neurocognitive Function, and Retinal Function. JAMA neurology. 2014 Aug 11.

[134] Bales KR, Verina T, Cummins DJ, Du Y, Dodel RC, Saura J, et al. Apolipoprotein E is essential for amyloid deposition in the APP(V717F) transgenic mouse model of Alz-heimer's disease. Proceedings of the National Academy of Sciences of the United States of America. 1999 Dec 21;96(26):15233-8.

[135] Kim J, Jiang H, Park S, Eltorai AE, Stewart FR, Yoon H, et al. Haploinsufficiency of human APOE reduces amyloid deposition in a mouse model of amyloid-beta amyloi-dosis. The Journal of neuroscience : the official journal of the Society for Neuro-science. 2011 Dec 7;31(49):18007-12.

[136] Bien-Ly N, Gillespie AK, Walker D, Yoon SY, Huang Y. Reducing human apolipo-protein E levels attenuates age-dependent Abeta accumulation in mutant human amyloid precursor protein transgenic mice. The Journal of neuroscience : the official journal of the Society for Neuroscience. 2012 Apr 4;32(14):4803-11.

[137] Holtzman DM, Fagan AM, Mackey B, Tenkova T, Sartorius L, Paul SM, et al. Apoli-poprotein E facilitates neuritic and cerebrovascular plaque formation in an Alzheim-er's disease model. Annals of neurology. 2000 Jun;47(6):739-47.

[138] Geschwind DH. Tau phosphorylation, tangles, and neurodegeneration: the chicken or the egg? Neuron. 2003 Oct 30;40(3):457-60.

[139] Brecht WJ, Harris FM, Chang S, Tesseur I, Yu GQ, Xu Q, et al. Neuron-specific apolipoprotein e4 proteolysis is associated with increased tau phosphorylation in brains of transgenic mice. The Journal of neuroscience : the official journal of the Society for Neuroscience. 2004 Mar 10;24(10):2527-34.

[140] Mahley RW, Huang Y. Apolipoprotein e sets the stage: response to injury triggers neuropathology. Neuron. 2012 Dec 6;76(5):871-85.

[141] Hamanaka H, Katoh-Fukui Y, Suzuki K, Kobayashi M, Suzuki R, Motegi Y, et al. Altered cholesterol metabolism in human apolipoprotein E4 knock-in mice. Human molecular genetics. 2000 Feb 12;9(3):353-61.

[142] Klein RC, Mace BE, Moore SD, Sullivan PM. Progressive loss of synaptic integrity in human apolipoprotein E4 targeted replacement mice and attenuation by apolipoprotein E2. Neuroscience. 2010 Dec 29;171(4):1265-72.

[143] Chen Y, Durakoglugil MS, Xian X, Herz J. ApoE4 reduces glutamate receptor function and synaptic plasticity by selectively impairing ApoE receptor recycling. Proceedings of the National Academy of Sciences of the United States of America. 2010 Jun 29;107(26):12011- 6.

[144] Alzheimer A, Stelzmann RA, Schnitzlein HN, Murtagh FR. An English translation of Alzheimer's 1907 paper, "Uber eine eigenartige Erkankung der Hirnrinde". Clinical anatomy. 1995;8(6):429-31.

[145] LaDu MJ, Shah JA, Reardon CA, Getz GS, Bu G, Hu J, et al. Apolipoprotein E and apolipoprotein E receptors modulate A beta-induced glial neuroinflammatory responses. Neurochemistry international. 2001 Nov-Dec;39(5-6):427-34.

[146] Pocivavsek A, Mikhailenko I, Strickland DK, Rebeck GW. Microglial low-density lipoprotein receptor-related protein 1 modulates c-Jun N-terminal kinase activation. Journal of neuroimmunology. 2009 Sep 29;214(1-2):25-32.

[147] Keene CD, Cudaback E, Li X, Montine KS, Montine TJ. Apolipoprotein E isoforms and regulation of the innate immune response in brain of patients with Alzheimer's disease. Current opinion in neurobiology. 2011 Dec;21(6):920-8.

[148] Grainger DJ, Reckless J, McKilligin E. Apolipoprotein E modulates clearance of apoptotic bodies in vitro and in vivo, resulting in a systemic proinflammatory state in apolipoprotein E-deficient mice. Journal of immunology. 2004 Nov 15;173(10): 6366-75.

[149] Lynch JR, Tang W, Wang H, Vitek MP, Bennett ER, Sullivan PM, et al. APOE genotype and an ApoE-mimetic peptide modify the systemic and central nervous system inflammatory response. The Journal of biological chemistry. 2003 Dec 5;278(49): 48529-33.

[150] Rodriguez GA, Tai LM, LaDu MJ, Rebeck GW. Human APOE4 increases microglia reactivity at Abeta plaques in a mouse model of Abeta deposition. Journal of neuro-inflammation. 2014;11:111.

[151] Zhu Y, Nwabuisi-Heath E, Dumanis SB, Tai LM, Yu C, Rebeck GW, et al. APOE genotype alters glial activation and loss of synaptic markers in mice. Glia. 2012 Apr; 60(4):559-69.

[152] Szekely CA, Breitner JC, Fitzpatrick AL, Rea TD, Psaty BM, Kuller LH, et al. NSAID use and dementia risk in the Cardiovascular Health Study: role of APOE and NSAID type. Neurology. 2008 Jan 1;70(1):17-24.

[153] Harold D, Abraham R, Hollingworth P, Sims R, Gerrish A, Hamshere ML, et al. Genome-wide association study identifies variants at CLU and PICALM associated with Alzheimer's disease. Nature genetics. 2009 Oct;41(10):1088-93.

[154] Lambert JC, Heath S, Even G, Campion D, Sleegers K, Hiltunen M, et al. Genome-wide association study identifies variants at CLU and CR1 associated with Alzheimer's disease. Nature genetics. 2009 Oct;41(10):1094-9.

[155] Jun G, Naj AC, Beecham GW, Wang LS, Buros J, Gallins PJ, et al. Meta-analysis confirms CR1, CLU, and PICALM as alzheimer disease risk loci and reveals interactions with APOE genotypes. Archives of neurology. 2010 Dec;67(12):1473-84.

[156] Mullan GM, McEneny J, Fuchs M, McMaster C, Todd S, McGuinness B, et al. Plasma clusterin levels and the rs11136000 genotype in individuals with mild cognitive impairment and Alzheimer's disease. Current Alzheimer research. 2013 Nov;10(9): 973-8.

[157] Thambisetty M, Simmons A, Velayudhan L, Hye A, Campbell J, Zhang Y, et al. Association of plasma clusterin concentration with severity, pathology, and progression in Alzheimer disease. Archives of general psychiatry. 2010 Jul;67(7):739-48.

[158] Schurmann B, Wiese B, Bickel H, Weyerer S, Riedel-Heller SG, Pentzek M, et al. Association of the Alzheimer's disease clusterin risk allele with plasma clusterin concentration. Journal of Alzheimer's disease : JAD. 2011;25(3):421-4.

[159] Braskie MN, Jahanshad N, Stein JL, Barysheva M, McMahon KL, de Zubicaray GI, et al. Common Alzheimer's disease risk variant within the CLU gene affects white matter microstructure in young adults. The Journal of neuroscience : the official journal of the Society for Neuroscience. 2011 May 4;31(18):6764-70.

[160] Erk S, Meyer-Lindenberg A, Opitz von Boberfeld C, Esslinger C, Schnell K, Kirsch P, et al. Hippocampal function in healthy carriers of the CLU Alzheimer's disease risk variant. The Journal of neuroscience : the official journal of the Society for Neuroscience. 2011 Dec 7;31(49):18180-4.

[161] Lancaster TM, Baird A, Wolf C, Jackson MC, Johnston SJ, Donev R, et al. Neural hyperactivation in carriers of the Alzheimer's risk variant on the clusterin gene. Europe-

an neuropsychopharmacology : the journal of the European College of Neuropsychopharmacology. 2011 Dec;21(12):880-4.

[162] Roussotte FF, Gutman BA, Madsen SK, Colby JB, Thompson PM, Alzheimer's Disease Neuroimaging I. Combined effects of Alzheimer risk variants in the CLU and ApoE genes on ventricular expansion patterns in the elderly. The Journal of neuroscience : the official journal of the Society for Neuroscience. 2014 May 7;34(19): 6537-45.

[163] Thambisetty M, Beason-Held LL, An Y, Kraut M, Nalls M, Hernandez DG, et al. Alzheimer risk variant CLU and brain function during aging. Biological psychiatry. 2013 Mar 1;73(5):399-405.

[164] Rodriguez-Rodriguez E, Sanchez-Juan P, Vazquez-Higuera JL, Mateo I, Pozueta A, Berciano J, et al. Genetic risk score predicting accelerated progression from mild cognitive impairment to Alzheimer's disease. Journal of neural transmission. 2013 May; 120(5):807-12.

[165] Elias-Sonnenschein LS, Helisalmi S, Natunen T, Hall A, Paajanen T, Herukka SK, et al. Genetic loci associated with Alzheimer's disease and cerebrospinal fluid biomarkers in a Finnish case-control cohort. PloS one. 2013;8(4):e59676.

[166] Kauwe JS, Cruchaga C, Karch CM, Sadler B, Lee M, Mayo K, et al. Fine mapping of genetic variants in BIN1, CLU, CR1 and PICALM for association with cerebrospinal fluid biomarkers for Alzheimer's disease. PloS one. 2011;6(2):e15918.

[167] Jongbloed W, Herrebout MA, Blankenstein MA, Veerhuis R. Quantification of clusterin in paired cerebrospinal fluid and plasma samples. Annals of clinical biochemistry. 2014 Sep;51(Pt 5):557-67.

[168] Desikan RS, Thompson WK, Holland D, Hess CP, Brewer JB, Zetterberg H, et al. The role of clusterin in amyloid-beta-associated neurodegeneration. JAMA neurology. 2014 Feb;71(2):180-7.

[169] Harr SD, Uint L, Hollister R, Hyman BT, Mendez AJ. Brain expression of apolipoproteins E, J, and A-I in Alzheimer's disease. Journal of neurochemistry. 1996 Jun;66(6): 2429-35.

[170] Nilselid AM, Davidsson P, Nagga K, Andreasen N, Fredman P, Blennow K. Clusterin in cerebrospinal fluid: analysis of carbohydrates and quantification of native and glycosylated forms. Neurochemistry international. 2006 Jun;48(8):718-28.

[171] Sihlbom C, Davidsson P, Sjogren M, Wahlund LO, Nilsson CL. Structural and quantitative comparison of cerebrospinal fluid glycoproteins in Alzheimer's disease patients and healthy individuals. Neurochemical research. 2008 Jul;33(7):1332-40.

[172] Baig S, Palmer LE, Owen MJ, Williams J, Kehoe PG, Love S. Clusterin mRNA and protein in Alzheimer's disease. Journal of Alzheimer's disease : JAD. 2012;28(2): 337-44.

[173] May PC, Johnson SA, Poirier J, Lampert-Etchells M, Finch CE. Altered gene expression in Alzheimer's disease brain tissue. The Canadian journal of neurological sciences Le journal canadien des sciences neurologiques. 1989 Nov;16(4 Suppl):473-6.

[174] Bertrand P, Poirier J, Oda T, Finch CE, Pasinetti GM. Association of apolipoprotein E genotype with brain levels of apolipoprotein E and apolipoprotein J (clusterin) in Alzheimer disease. Brain research Molecular brain research. 1995 Oct;33(1):174-8.

[175] Chen LH, Kao PY, Fan YH, Ho DT, Chan CS, Yik PY, et al. Polymorphisms of CR1, CLU and PICALM confer susceptibility of Alzheimer's disease in a southern Chinese population. Neurobiology of aging. 2012 Jan;33(1):210 e1-7.

[176] Lidstrom AM, Bogdanovic N, Hesse C, Volkman I, Davidsson P, Blennow K. Clusterin (apolipoprotein J) protein levels are increased in hippocampus and in frontal cortex in Alzheimer's disease. Experimental neurology. 1998 Dec;154(2):511-21.

[177] Oda T, Pasinetti GM, Osterburg HH, Anderson C, Johnson SA, Finch CE. Purification and characterization of brain clusterin. Biochemical and biophysical research communications. 1994 Nov 15;204(3):1131-6.

[178] Martin-Rehrmann MD, Hoe HS, Capuani EM, Rebeck GW. Association of apolipoprotein J-positive beta-amyloid plaques with dystrophic neurites in Alzheimer's disease brain. Neurotoxicity research. 2005;7(3):231-42.

[179] McGeer PL, Kawamata T, Walker DG. Distribution of clusterin in Alzheimer brain tissue. Brain research. 1992 May 8;579(2):337-41.

[180] Howlett DR, Hortobagyi T, Francis PT. Clusterin associates specifically with Abeta40 in Alzheimer's disease brain tissue. Brain pathology. 2013 Nov;23(6):623-32.

[181] Kida S, Weller RO, Zhang ET, Phillips MJ, Iannotti F. Anatomical pathways for lymphatic drainage of the brain and their pathological significance. Neuropathology and applied neurobiology. 1995 Jun;21(3):181-4.

[182] Hughes TM, Lopez OL, Evans RW, Kamboh MI, Williamson JD, Klunk WE, et al. Markers of cholesterol transport are associated with amyloid deposition in the brain. Neurobiology of aging. 2014 Apr;35(4):802-7.

[183] Silajdzic E, Minthon L, Bjorkqvist M, Hansson O. No diagnostic value of plasma clusterin in Alzheimer's disease. PloS one. 2012;7(11):e50237.

[184] Thambisetty M, An Y, Kinsey A, Koka D, Saleem M, Guntert A, et al. Plasma clusterin concentration is associated with longitudinal brain atrophy in mild cognitive impairment. NeuroImage. 2012 Jan 2;59(1):212-7.

[185] L IJ, Dekker LJ, Koudstaal PJ, Hofman A, Sillevis Smitt PA, Breteler MM, et al. Serum clusterin levels are not increased in presymptomatic Alzheimer's disease. Journal of proteome research. 2011 Apr 1;10(4):2006-10.

[186] Hye A, Riddoch-Contreras J, Baird AL, Ashton NJ, Bazenet C, Leung R, et al. Plasma proteins predict conversion to dementia from prodromal disease. Alzheimer's & dementia : the journal of the Alzheimer's Association. 2014 Jul 3.

[187] Schrijvers EM, Koudstaal PJ, Hofman A, Breteler MM. Plasma clusterin and the risk of Alzheimer disease. Jama. 2011 Apr 6;305(13):1322-6.

[188] Thambisetty M. Do extracellular chaperone proteins in plasma have potential as Alzheimer's disease biomarkers? Biomarkers in medicine. 2010 Dec;4(6):831-4.

[189] DeMattos RB, O'Dell M A, Parsadanian M, Taylor JW, Harmony JA, Bales KR, et al. Clusterin promotes amyloid plaque formation and is critical for neuritic toxicity in a mouse model of Alzheimer's disease. Proceedings of the National Academy of Sciences of the United States of America. 2002 Aug 6;99(16):10843-8.

[190] Mulder SD, Nielsen HM, Blankenstein MA, Eikelenboom P, Veerhuis R. Apolipoproteins E and J interfere with amyloid-beta uptake by primary human astrocytes and microglia in vitro. Glia. 2014 Apr;62(4):493-503.

[191] Killick R, Ribe EM, Al-Shawi R, Malik B, Hooper C, Fernandes C, et al. Clusterin regulates beta-amyloid toxicity via Dickkopf-1-driven induction of the wnt-PCP-JNK pathway. Molecular psychiatry. 2014 Jan;19(1):88-98.

[192] Bell RD, Sagare AP, Friedman AE, Bedi GS, Holtzman DM, Deane R, et al. Transport pathways for clearance of human Alzheimer's amyloid beta-peptide and apolipoproteins E and J in the mouse central nervous system. Journal of cerebral blood flow and metabolism : official journal of the International Society of Cerebral Blood Flow and Metabolism. 2007 May;27(5):909-18.

[193] Narayan P, Meehan S, Carver JA, Wilson MR, Dobson CM, Klenerman D. Amyloid-beta oligomers are sequestered by both intracellular and extracellular chaperones. Biochemistry. 2012 Nov 20;51(46):9270-6.

[194] Saczynski JS, White L, Peila RL, Rodriguez BL, Launer LJ. The relation between apolipoprotein A-I and dementia: the Honolulu-Asia aging study. American journal of epidemiology. 2007 May 1;165(9):985-92.

[195] Reitz C, Tang MX, Schupf N, Manly JJ, Mayeux R, Luchsinger JA. Association of higher levels of high-density lipoprotein cholesterol in elderly individuals and lower risk of late-onset Alzheimer disease. Archives of neurology. 2010 Dec;67(12):1491-7.

[196] Reed B, Villeneuve S, Mack W, DeCarli C, Chui HC, Jagust W. Associations between serum cholesterol levels and cerebral amyloidosis. JAMA neurology. 2014 Feb;71(2): 195- 200.

[197] Kawano M, Kawakami M, Otsuka M, Yashima H, Yaginuma T, Ueki A. Marked decrease of plasma apolipoprotein AI and AII in Japanese patients with late-onset non-familial Alzheimer's disease. Clinica chimica acta; international journal of clinical chemistry. 1995 Aug 14;239(2):209-11.

[198]   Kuriyama M, Takahashi K, Yamano T, Hokezu Y, Togo S, Osame M, et al. Low levels of serum apolipoprotein A I and A II in senile dementia. The Japanese journal of psychiatry and neurology. 1994 Sep;48(3):589-93.

[199]   Shih YH, Tsai KJ, Lee CW, Shiesh SC, Chen WT, Pai MC, et al. Apolipoprotein C-III is an Amyloid-beta-Binding Protein and an Early Marker for Alzheimer's Disease. Journal of Alzheimer's disease : JAD. 2014 Mar 31.

[200]   Merched A, Xia Y, Visvikis S, Serot JM, Siest G. Decreased high-density lipoprotein cholesterol and serum apolipoprotein AI concentrations are highly correlated with the severity of Alzheimer's disease. Neurobiology of aging. 2000 Jan-Feb;21(1):27-30.

[201]   Castano EM, Roher AE, Esh CL, Kokjohn TA, Beach T. Comparative proteomics of cerebrospinal fluid in neuropathologically-confirmed Alzheimer's disease and non-demented elderly subjects. Neurological research. 2006 Mar;28(2):155-63.

[202]   Song H, Saito K, Seishima M, Noma A, Urakami K, Nakashima K. Cerebrospinal fluid apo E and apo A-I concentrations in early- and late-onset Alzheimer's disease. Neuroscience letters. 1997 Aug 15;231(3):175-8.

[203]   Lefterov I, Fitz NF, Cronican AA, Fogg A, Lefterov P, Kodali R, et al. Apolipoprotein A-I deficiency increases cerebral amyloid angiopathy and cognitive deficits in APP/PS1DeltaE9 mice. The Journal of biological chemistry. 2010 Nov 19;285(47):36945-57.

[204]   Lewis TL, Cao D, Lu H, Mans RA, Su YR, Jungbauer L, et al. Overexpression of human apolipoprotein A-I preserves cognitive function and attenuates neuroinflammation and cerebral amyloid angiopathy in a mouse model of Alzheimer disease. The Journal of biological chemistry. 2010 Nov 19;285(47):36958-68.

[205]   de Magalhaes JP, Curado J, Church GM. Meta-analysis of age-related gene expression profiles identifies common signatures of aging. Bioinformatics. 2009 Apr 1;25(7):875-81.

[206]   Terrisse L, Poirier J, Bertrand P, Merched A, Visvikis S, Siest G, et al. Increased levels of apolipoprotein D in cerebrospinal fluid and hippocampus of Alzheimer's patients. Journal of neurochemistry. 1998 Oct;71(4):1643-50.

[207]   Glockner F, Ohm TG. Hippocampal apolipoprotein D level depends on Braak stage and APOE genotype. Neuroscience. 2003;122(1):103-10.

[208]   Abildayeva K, Berbee JF, Blokland A, Jansen PJ, Hoek FJ, Meijer O, et al. Human apolipoprotein C-I expression in mice impairs learning and memory functions. Journal of lipid research. 2008 Apr;49(4):856-69.

[209]   Cudaback E, Li X, Yang Y, Yoo T, Montine KS, Craft S, et al. Apolipoprotein C-I is an APOE genotype-dependent suppressor of glial activation. Journal of neuroinflammation. 2012;9:192.

[210] Poduslo SE, Neal M, Herring K, Shelly J. The apolipoprotein CI A allele as a risk factor for Alzheimer's disease. Neurochemical research. 1998 Mar;23(3):361-7.

[211] Drigalenko E, Poduslo S, Elston R. Interaction of the apolipoprotein E and CI loci in predisposing to late-onset Alzheimer's disease. Neurology. 1998 Jul;51(1):131-5.

[212] Csaszar A, Kalman J, Szalai C, Janka Z, Romics L. Association of the apolipoprotein A-IV codon 360 mutation in patients with Alzheimer's disease. Neuroscience letters. 1997 Jul 25;230(3):151-4.

[213] Cui Y, Huang M, He Y, Zhang S, Luo Y. Genetic ablation of apolipoprotein A-IV accelerates Alzheimer's disease pathogenesis in a mouse model. The American journal of pathology. 2011 Mar;178(3):1298-308.

[214] Shih YH, Tsai KJ, Lee CW, Shiesh SC, Chen WT, Pai MC, et al. Apolipoprotein C-III is an amyloid-beta-binding protein and an early marker for Alzheimer's disease. Journal of Alzheimer's disease : JAD. 2014;41(3):855-65.

[215] Pahnke J, Langer O, Krohn M. Alzheimer's and ABC transporters - new opportunities for diagnostics and treatment. Neurobiology of disease. 2014 Apr 16.

[216] Koldamova R, Fitz NF, Lefterov I. ATP-binding cassette transporter A1: From metabolism to neurodegeneration. Neurobiology of disease. 2014 May 17.

[217] Hirsch-Reinshagen V, Maia LF, Burgess BL, Blain JF, Naus KE, McIsaac SA, et al. The absence of ABCA1 decreases soluble ApoE levels but does not diminish amyloid deposition in two murine models of Alzheimer disease. The Journal of biological chemistry. 2005 Dec 30;280(52):43243-56.

[218] Wahrle SE, Jiang H, Parsadanian M, Hartman RE, Bales KR, Paul SM, et al. Deletion of Abca1 increases Abeta deposition in the PDAPP transgenic mouse model of Alzheimer disease. The Journal of biological chemistry. 2005 Dec 30;280(52):43236-42.

[219] Koldamova R, Staufenbiel M, Lefterov I. Lack of ABCA1 considerably decreases brain ApoE level and increases amyloid deposition in APP23 mice. The Journal of biological chemistry. 2005 Dec 30;280(52):43224-35.

[220] Lefterov I, Fitz NF, Cronican A, Lefterov P, Staufenbiel M, Koldamova R. Memory deficits in APP23/Abca1+/- mice correlate with the level of Abeta oligomers. ASN neuro. 2009;1(2).

[221] Fitz NF, Cronican AA, Saleem M, Fauq AH, Chapman R, Lefterov I, et al. Abca1 deficiency affects Alzheimer's disease-like phenotype in human ApoE4 but not in ApoE3- targeted replacement mice. The Journal of neuroscience : the official journal of the Society for Neuroscience. 2012 Sep 19;32(38):13125-36.

[222] Lefterov I, Bookout A, Wang Z, Staufenbiel M, Mangelsdorf D, Koldamova R. Expression profiling in APP23 mouse brain: inhibition of Abeta amyloidosis and in-

flammation in response to LXR agonist treatment. Molecular neurodegeneration. 2007;2:20.

[223] Koldamova RP, Lefterov IM, Staufenbiel M, Wolfe D, Huang S, Glorioso JC, et al. The liver X receptor ligand T0901317 decreases amyloid beta production in vitro and in a mouse model of Alzheimer's disease. The Journal of biological chemistry. 2005 Feb 11;280(6):4079-88.

[224] Riddell DR, Zhou H, Comery TA, Kouranova E, Lo CF, Warwick HK, et al. The LXR agonist TO901317 selectively lowers hippocampal Abeta42 and improves memory in the Tg2576 mouse model of Alzheimer's disease. Molecular and cellular neurosciences. 2007 Apr;34(4):621-8.

[225] Jiang Q, Lee CY, Mandrekar S, Wilkinson B, Cramer P, Zelcer N, et al. ApoE promotes the proteolytic degradation of Abeta. Neuron. 2008 Jun 12;58(5):681-93.

[226] Fitz NF, Cronican A, Pham T, Fogg A, Fauq AH, Chapman R, et al. Liver X receptor agonist treatment ameliorates amyloid pathology and memory deficits caused by high-fat diet in APP23 mice. The Journal of neuroscience : the official journal of the Society for Neuroscience. 2010 May 19;30(20):6862-72.

[227] Cramer PE, Cirrito JR, Wesson DW, Lee CY, Karlo JC, Zinn AE, et al. ApoE-directed therapeutics rapidly clear beta-amyloid and reverse deficits in AD mouse models. Science. 2012 Mar 23;335(6075):1503-6.

[228] Vanmierlo T, Rutten K, Dederen J, Bloks VW, van Vark-van der Zee LC, Kuipers F, et al. Liver X receptor activation restores memory in aged AD mice without reducing amyloid. Neurobiology of aging. 2011 Jul;32(7):1262-72.

[229] Donkin JJ, Stukas S, Hirsch-Reinshagen V, Namjoshi D, Wilkinson A, May S, et al. ATP-binding cassette transporter A1 mediates the beneficial effects of the liver X receptor agonist GW3965 on object recognition memory and amyloid burden in amyloid precursor protein/presenilin 1 mice. The Journal of biological chemistry. 2010 Oct 29;285(44):34144- 54.

[230] Fitz NF, Castranio EL, Carter AY, Kodali R, Lefterov I, Koldamova R. Improvement of Memory Deficits and Amyloid-beta Clearance in Aged APP23 Mice Treated with a Combination of Anti-Amyloid-beta Antibody and LXR Agonist. Journal of Alzheimer's disease: JAD. 2014 Mar 18.

[231] Fitz NF, Cronican AA, Lefterov I, Koldamova R. Comment on "ApoE-directed therapeutics rapidly clear beta-amyloid and reverse deficits in AD mouse models". Science. 2013 May 24;340(6135):924-c.

[232] Tesseur I, Lo AC, Roberfroid A, Dietvorst S, Van Broeck B, Borgers M, et al. Comment on "ApoE-directed therapeutics rapidly clear beta-amyloid and reverse deficits in AD mouse models". Science. 2013 May 24;340(6135):924-e.

[233] Wang XF, Cao YW, Feng ZZ, Fu D, Ma YS, Zhang F, et al. Quantitative assessment of the effect of ABCA1 gene polymorphism on the risk of Alzheimer's disease. Molecular biology reports. 2013 Feb;40(2):779-85.

[234] Frikke-Schmidt R, Nordestgaard BG, Stene MC, Sethi AA, Remaley AT, Schnohr P, et al. Association of loss-of-function mutations in the ABCA1 gene with high-density lipoprotein cholesterol levels and risk of ischemic heart disease. Jama. 2008 Jun 4;299(21):2524-32.

[235] Clee SM, Kastelein JJ, van Dam M, Marcil M, Roomp K, Zwarts KY, et al. Age and residual cholesterol efflux affect HDL cholesterol levels and coronary artery disease in ABCA1 heterozygotes. The Journal of clinical investigation. 2000 Nov;106(10): 1263-70.

[236] Rader DJ, deGoma EM. Approach to the patient with extremely low HDL-cholesterol. The Journal of clinical endocrinology and metabolism. 2012 Oct;97(10):3399-407.

[237] Naj AC, Jun G, Beecham GW, Wang LS, Vardarajan BN, Buros J, et al. Common variants at MS4A4/MS4A6E, CD2AP, CD33 and EPHA1 are associated with late-onset Alzheimer's disease. Nature genetics. 2011 May;43(5):436-41.

[238] Allen M, Zou F, Chai HS, Younkin CS, Crook J, Pankratz VS, et al. Novel late-onset Alzheimer disease loci variants associate with brain gene expression. Neurology. 2012 Jul 17;79(3):221-8.

[239] Karch CM, Jeng AT, Nowotny P, Cady J, Cruchaga C, Goate AM. Expression of novel Alzheimer's disease risk genes in control and Alzheimer's disease brains. PloS one. 2012;7(11):e50976.

[240] Reitz C, Jun G, Naj A, Rajbhandary R, Vardarajan BN, Wang LS, et al. Variants in the ATP-binding cassette transporter (ABCA7), apolipoprotein E 4,and the risk of late-onset Alzheimer disease in African Americans. Jama. 2013 Apr 10;309(14):1483-92.

[241] Vasquez JB, Fardo DW, Estus S. ABCA7 expression is associated with Alzheimer's disease polymorphism and disease status. Neuroscience letters. 2013 Nov 27;556:58-62.

[242] Shulman JM, Chen K, Keenan BT, Chibnik LB, Fleisher A, Thiyyagura P, et al. Genetic susceptibility for Alzheimer disease neuritic plaque pathology. JAMA neurology. 2013 Sep 1;70(9):1150-7.

[243] Beecham GW, Hamilton K, Naj AC, Martin ER, Huentelman M, Myers AJ, et al. Genome-Wide Association Meta-analysis of Neuropathologic Features of Alzheimer's Disease and Related Dementias. PLoS genetics. 2014 Sep;10(9):e1004606.

[244] Hollingworth P, Harold D, Sims R, Gerrish A, Lambert JC, Carrasquillo MM, et al. Common variants at ABCA7, MS4A6A/MS4A4E, EPHA1, CD33 and CD2AP are associated with Alzheimer's disease. Nature genetics. 2011 May;43(5):429-35.

[245] Kim WS, Li H, Ruberu K, Chan S, Elliott DA, Low JK, et al. Deletion of Abca7 increases cerebral amyloid-beta accumulation in the J20 mouse model of Alzheimer's disease. The Journal of neuroscience : the official journal of the Society for Neuroscience. 2013 Mar 6;33(10):4387-94.

[246] Burgess BL, Parkinson PF, Racke MM, Hirsch-Reinshagen V, Fan J, Wong C, et al. ABCG1 influences the brain cholesterol biosynthetic pathway but does not affect amyloid precursor protein or apolipoprotein E metabolism in vivo. Journal of lipid research. 2008 Jun;49(6):1254-67.

[247] Rousset X, Shamburek R, Vaisman B, Amar M, Remaley AT. Lecithin cholesterol acyltransferase: an anti- or pro-atherogenic factor? Current atherosclerosis reports. 2011 Jun;13(3):249-56.

[248] Desrumaux C, Pisoni A, Meunier J, Deckert V, Athias A, Perrier V, et al. Increased amyloid-beta peptide-induced memory deficits in phospholipid transfer protein (PLTP) gene knockout mice. Neuropsychopharmacology : official publication of the American College of Neuropsychopharmacology. 2013 Apr;38(5):817-25.

[249] Wang H, Yu Y, Chen W, Cui Y, Luo T, Ma J, et al. PLTP deficiency impairs learning and memory capabilities partially due to alteration of amyloid-beta metabolism in old mice. Journal of Alzheimer's disease : JAD. 2014;39(1):79-88.

[250] Arias-Vasquez A, Isaacs A, Aulchenko YS, Hofman A, Oostra BA, Breteler M, et al. The cholesteryl ester transfer protein (CETP) gene and the risk of Alzheimer's disease. Neurogenetics. 2007 Aug;8(3):189-93.

[251] Barzilai N, Atzmon G, Schechter C, Schaefer EJ, Cupples AL, Lipton R, et al. Unique lipoprotein phenotype and genotype associated with exceptional longevity. Jama. 2003 Oct 15;290(15):2030-40.

[252] Cellini E, Nacmias B, Olivieri F, Ortenzi L, Tedde A, Bagnoli S, et al. Cholesteryl ester transfer protein (CETP) I405V polymorphism and longevity in Italian centenarians. Mechanisms of ageing and development. 2005 Jun-Jul;126(6-7):826-8.

[253] Li Q, Huang P, He QC, Lin QZ, Wu J, Yin RX. Association between the CETP polymorphisms and the risk of Alzheimer's disease, carotid atherosclerosis, longevity, and the efficacy of statin therapy. Neurobiology of aging. 2014 Jun;35(6):1513 e13-23.

[254] Novelli V, Viviani Anselmi C, Roncarati R, Guffanti G, Malovini A, Piluso G, et al. Lack of replication of genetic associations with human longevity. Biogerontology. 2008 Apr;9(2):85-92.

[255] Sun L, Hu CY, Shi XH, Zheng CG, Huang ZZ, Lv ZP, et al. Trans-ethnical shift of the risk genotype in the CETP I405V with longevity: a Chinese case-control study and meta- analysis. PloS one. 2013;8(8):e72537.

[256] Yang JK, Gong YY, Xie L, Yang Y, Xu LY, Zhang YP. Association study of promoter polymorphisms in the CETP gene with longevity in the Han Chinese population. Molecular biology reports. 2014 Jan;41(1):325-9.

[257] Warstadt NM, Dennis EL, Jahanshad N, Kohannim O, Nir TM, McMahon KL, et al. Serum cholesterol and variant in cholesterol-related gene CETP predict white matter microstructure. Neurobiology of aging. 2014 Nov;35(11):2504-13.

[258] Rodriguez E, Mateo I, Infante J, Llorca J, Berciano J, Combarros O. Cholesteryl ester transfer protein (CETP) polymorphism modifies the Alzheimer's disease risk associated with APOE epsilon4 allele. Journal of neurology. 2006 Feb;253(2):181-5.

[259] Chen Y, Jia L, Wei C, Wang F, Lv H, Jia J. Association between polymorphisms in the apolipoprotein D gene and sporadic Alzheimer's disease. Brain research. 2008 Oct 3;1233:196-202.

[260] Murphy EA, Roddey JC, McEvoy LK, Holland D, Hagler DJ, Jr., Dale AM, et al. CETP polymorphisms associate with brain structure, atrophy rate, and Alzheimer's disease risk in an APOE-dependent manner. Brain imaging and behavior. 2012 Mar; 6(1):16-26.

[261] Sanders AE, Wang C, Katz M, Derby CA, Barzilai N, Ozelius L, et al. Association of a functional polymorphism in the cholesteryl ester transfer protein (CETP) gene with memory decline and incidence of dementia. Jama. 2010 Jan 13;303(2):150-8.

[262] Deane R, Wu Z, Sagare A, Davis J, Du Yan S, Hamm K, et al. LRP/amyloid beta- peptide interaction mediates differential brain efflux of Abeta isoforms. Neuron. 2004 Aug 5;43(3):333-44.

[263] Kanekiyo T, Cirrito JR, Liu CC, Shinohara M, Li J, Schuler DR, et al. Neuronal clearance of amyloid-beta by endocytic receptor LRP1. The Journal of neuroscience : the official journal of the Society for Neuroscience. 2013 Dec 4;33(49):19276-83.

[264] Shibata M, Yamada S, Kumar SR, Calero M, Bading J, Frangione B, et al. Clearance of Alzheimer's amyloid-ss(1-40) peptide from brain by LDL receptor-related protein-1 at the blood-brain barrier. The Journal of clinical investigation. 2000 Dec;106(12): 1489-99.

[265] Tamamizu-Kato S, Cohen JK, Drake CB, Kosaraju MG, Drury J, Narayanaswami V. Interaction with amyloid beta peptide compromises the lipid binding function of apolipoprotein E. Biochemistry. 2008 May 6;47(18):5225-34.

[266] Van Uden E, Mallory M, Veinbergs I, Alford M, Rockenstein E, Masliah E. Increased extracellular amyloid deposition and neurodegeneration in human amyloid precursor protein transgenic mice deficient in receptor-associated protein. The Journal of neuroscience : the official journal of the Society for Neuroscience. 2002 Nov 1;22(21): 9298-304.

[267] Deane R, Sagare A, Hamm K, Parisi M, Lane S, Finn MB, et al. apoE isoform-specific disruption of amyloid beta peptide clearance from mouse brain. The Journal of clinical investigation. 2008 Dec;118(12):4002-13.

[268] Cao D, Fukuchi K, Wan H, Kim H, Li L. Lack of LDL receptor aggravates learning deficits and amyloid deposits in Alzheimer transgenic mice. Neurobiology of aging. 2006 Nov;27(11):1632-43.

[269] Castellano JM, Deane R, Gottesdiener AJ, Verghese PB, Stewart FR, West T, et al. Low-density lipoprotein receptor overexpression enhances the rate of brain-to-blood Abeta clearance in a mouse model of beta-amyloidosis. Proceedings of the National Academy of Sciences of the United States of America. 2012 Sep 18;109(38):15502-7.

[270] Beffert U, Morfini G, Bock HH, Reyna H, Brady ST, Herz J. Reelin-mediated signaling locally regulates protein kinase B/Akt and glycogen synthase kinase 3beta. The Journal of biological chemistry. 2002 Dec 20;277(51):49958-64.

[271] Ohkubo N, Lee YD, Morishima A, Terashima T, Kikkawa S, Tohyama M, et al. Apolipoprotein E and Reelin ligands modulate tau phosphorylation through an apolipoprotein E receptor/disabled-1/glycogen synthase kinase-3beta cascade. FASEB journal : official publication of the Federation of American Societies for Experimental Biology. 2003 Feb;17(2):295-7.

[272] Ridker PM. LDL cholesterol: controversies and future therapeutic directions. Lancet. 2014 Aug 16;384(9943):607-17.

[273] Beffert U, Arguin C, Poirier J. The polymorphism in exon 3 of the low density lipoprotein receptor-related protein gene is weakly associated with Alzheimer's disease. Neuroscience letters. 1999 Jan 4;259(1):29-32.

[274] Sanchez-Guerra M, Combarros O, Infante J, Llorca J, Berciano J, Fontalba A, et al. Case-control study and meta-analysis of low density lipoprotein receptor-related protein gene exon 3 polymorphism in Alzheimer's disease. Neuroscience letters. 2001 Dec 4;316(1):17-20.

[275] Vazquez-Higuera JL, Mateo I, Sanchez-Juan P, Rodriguez-Rodriguez E, Pozueta A, Infante J, et al. Genetic interaction between tau and the apolipoprotein E receptor LRP1 Increases Alzheimer's disease risk. Dementia and geriatric cognitive disorders. 2009;28(2):116-20.

[276] Vargas T, Bullido MJ, Martinez-Garcia A, Antequera D, Clarimon J, Rosich-Estrago M, et al. A megalin polymorphism associated with promoter activity and Alzheimer's disease risk. American journal of medical genetics Part B, Neuropsychiatric genetics : the official publication of the International Society of Psychiatric Genetics. 2010 Jun 5;153B(4):895-902.

[277] Wang LL, Pan XL, Wang Y, Tang HD, Deng YL, Ren RJ, et al. A single nucleotide polymorphism in LRP2 is associated with susceptibility to Alzheimer's disease in the

Chinese population. Clinica chimica acta; international journal of clinical chemistry. 2011 Jan 30;412(3-4):268-70.

[278] Miyashita A, Koike A, Jun G, Wang LS, Takahashi S, Matsubara E, et al. SORL1 is genetically associated with late-onset Alzheimer's disease in Japanese, Koreans and Caucasians. PloS one. 2013;8(4):e58618.

[279] Rogaeva E, Meng Y, Lee JH, Gu Y, Kawarai T, Zou F, et al. The neuronal sortilin- related receptor SORL1 is genetically associated with Alzheimer disease. Nature genetics. 2007 Feb;39(2):168-77.

[280] Scherzer CR, Offe K, Gearing M, Rees HD, Fang G, Heilman CJ, et al. Loss of apolipoprotein E receptor LR11 in Alzheimer disease. Archives of neurology. 2004 Aug; 61(8):1200-5.

[281] Felsky D, Szeszko P, Yu L, Honer WG, De Jager PL, Schneider JA, et al. The SORL1 gene and convergent neural risk for Alzheimer's disease across the human lifespan. Molecular psychiatry. 2013 Oct 29.

3

Epidemiology of Alzheimer's Disease with the Projection of Falls Among the Aged Population

Aysegul Uludag, Sibel Cevizci and Ahmet Uludag

Additional information is available at the end of the chapter

1. Introduction

With aging, the loss of the ability to adapt to environmental factors in progressive decline occurs. Particularly in North European countries, the elderly population continues to gradually increase. Currently, in developing countries with a high youth population,it has been mentioned that the size of epidemiology in the aging population revealed a more realistic projection. The aging population is rapidly increasing. Of the 600 million elderly (60 years and over) that are living,the ratio will increase by 25% in the next 25 years, and the population of over 65 years old is expected to increase by 88% in the world. Most of the older population is found in developed countries than that are indicated. In this projection, the determination of health policies for the elderly necessarily becomes a first priority.

The old age period needs to be examined in physical, psychological, and social aspects. While physical changes occur in a chronological order, psychological perception changes are observed in learning, psychomotor, and personality characteristics. In the aspect of social perspective, the people live in many limitations [1]. The elderly population suffer with the following: approximately 8.0% have serious cognitive problems; 20% have chronic diseases, vision problems, and hearing loss; and 33% live with a limitation on movements [2].

Dementia is defined as one of the biggest problems faced by the elderly population. It is an overall term for diseases and conditions characterized by a decline in memory or other thinking skills that affects a person's ability to perform daily activities. According to DSM V criteria, dementia can be defined as a major and mild neurocognitive disorders. In epidemiological data, 24.2 million people live with dementia at that time, with 4.6 million new cases arising every year [3]. Dementia increases with age, especially over the age of 65 which are 1.5 times more often seen. Many conditions may cause dementia. However, the Alzheimer's disease (AD) is one of the reasons of the dementia that estimates 60-80%.

Alzheimer's disease is defined as a progressive loss of the cognitive function. This function loss history starts with the loss of memory and function, and eventually to all the intellectual activities of daily living and leads to premature death. Beta-amyloid plaques, neurofibrillary tangles, and neurodegeneration are the hallmark pathologic characteristics of AD [4]. To establish a diagnosis of AD with the onset of symptoms that can be done, in fact, already started the beginning of the 20 year before. Etiology has not been fully clarified, but the underlying causes are genetics, age, family history, the Apolipoprotein E-ε4 gene (APOE-ε4), mild cognitive impairment, education level, traumatic brain injury, and cardiovascular risk factors [5].

Alzheimer's disease causes slowly progressive irreversible cognitive destruction with the loss of performing even the daily activities. In particular, the most common problems encountered in this process is falling. Falls in patients have clinically more severe chronic process and present additional morbidity while mortality is increases. Alzheimer's disease has approximately 2 times higher risk for falling [6,7]. For patients with dementia, when they fall, they are three times more likely to have broken hips. Hip fracture further increase the death rate of AD patients [8]. In AD patients, increased risk of falling remains less understood. In studies, cerebral white matter lesions may relate to cognition and postural balance [9-10].

In this chapter, the epidemiology of Alzheimer's Disease with etiologic factors will be discussed, and with this projection, the risk and importance of falls in these patients will also be tackled.

2. The aging population

With aging, loss of the ability to adapt to environmental factors in progressive decline and aging population is rapidly increasing. Of 600 million elderly (60 years and over) that are living, the ratio will increase by 25% in the next 25 years, and the 65+ population is expected to increase by 88% in the world. Most of the older population is found in developed countries than that are indicated. In the year of 2056, 29.5% of Canadians, which is roughly 10.5 million people, are expected to be above 65 years of age [11]. Approximately 8% of the elderly population live with serious cognitive problems, while 20% have chronic diseases, vision problems, and hearing loss, while the another 33% live with limitation of movements [2,12].

While the geriatric population increases, the incidence of chronic diseases also increases. In particular, there are many physiological changes that occur in the geriatric period. The most prominent of these occur in the skeletal system. With aging, bone resorption decreases and senile osteoporosis occurs. In women, the menopause accelerated osteoporosis, and it threatens both male and female with aging. In addition to this change in the geriatric period, gastrointestinal system changes occur that reduce appetite and prevent the absorption of nutrients. This process in the geriatric period affects both the dementia process as well as increase the risk of co-morbidity.

There are also social aspects of geriatric patients with the same changes. The most prominent of these is related to the loss of spouse or loss of family members. Work situations, such as separation or lack of income increases, results to social problems in the elderly.

Today, in developed countries live alone in geriatric period stood out, with the rise of industrialization. In developing countries geriatrics are also dwindling along with family members. This facilitates the social isolation occuring in the aging population that live on their own.

One of the most significant changes experienced by the geriatric age group is also a change in mental health. Especially due to social isolation or existing health problems, mood disorders in the geriatric population is emerging. At the inital stage of dementia in people with mood changes, it is difficult to recognize the coexistence of disorder or delay.

3. The aging population and falls

In the elderly, physiologically changes and many chronic diseases occur, and the geriatric population also experience comorbidity problems. Falling is one of the major problems causing the increasing comorbidities and mortality rates. Falls, in the geriatric population, is the fifth leading cause of mortality [13]. Every year, geriatric patients aged 65 years and over is reduced by 30%, and for patients over 85 years of age, by 50%. Each year, 30-50% of falls are in nursing homes and 40% of those individuals fall again [14].

In the study from South Asia, it was found that the incidence of falls in China was 6-31%, while in Japan, it was 20% [15-17]. According to the WHO report, the rate of hospital admission caused by falls was found to be 1.6 to 3.0 per 10,000 population for people at the aged 60 years and over in Australia, Canada, the United Kingdom of Great Britain, and Northern Ireland (UK) [15]. Forty percent of all injury deaths are caused by falls [18]. Populations have various fall fatality rate for people aged 65 years and over: in the USA, 36.8 per 100,000 population; in Canada, 9.4; in Finland, 55.4 for people aged 50 and over [19-21]. Figure 1 indicates fatal falls by age group and gender [15,22]. Fatal fall rates increase with age for both gender, and the highest rate is seen at the age of 85 years and over. It has been found that men reported poorer health and a greater number of underlying conditions than women. These include increasing hip fracture and the risk of mortality [23].

Although population ageing is a triumph of humanity related to the extension of life-span, it brings back some challenges for societies [24]. The absolute number of people aged 60 years and over is expected to increase from 688 million in 2006 to 2 billion by 2050. For the first time, the population of aged people will be greater than the population of children under the 14 years of age [15]. In addition, being predisposed to falls and its serious consequences is fastest growing at the age of 80 and over. Figure 2 shows the population pyramid in 2005 and 2025 [15]. This figure shows that the percentage of older population is growing in parallel with a decreasing percentage of the younger population. The triangular shape of the 2005 population pyramid will transform into the more cylinder-like form in 2025 [15].

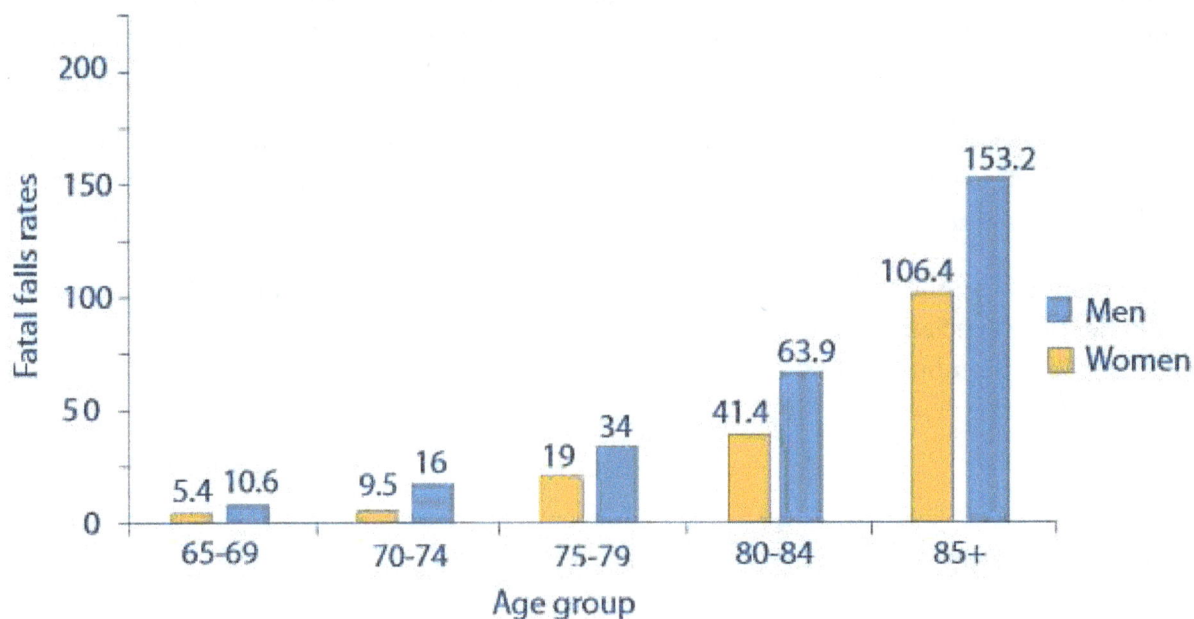

Figure 1. Fatal fall rates by age and sex group[15,22].

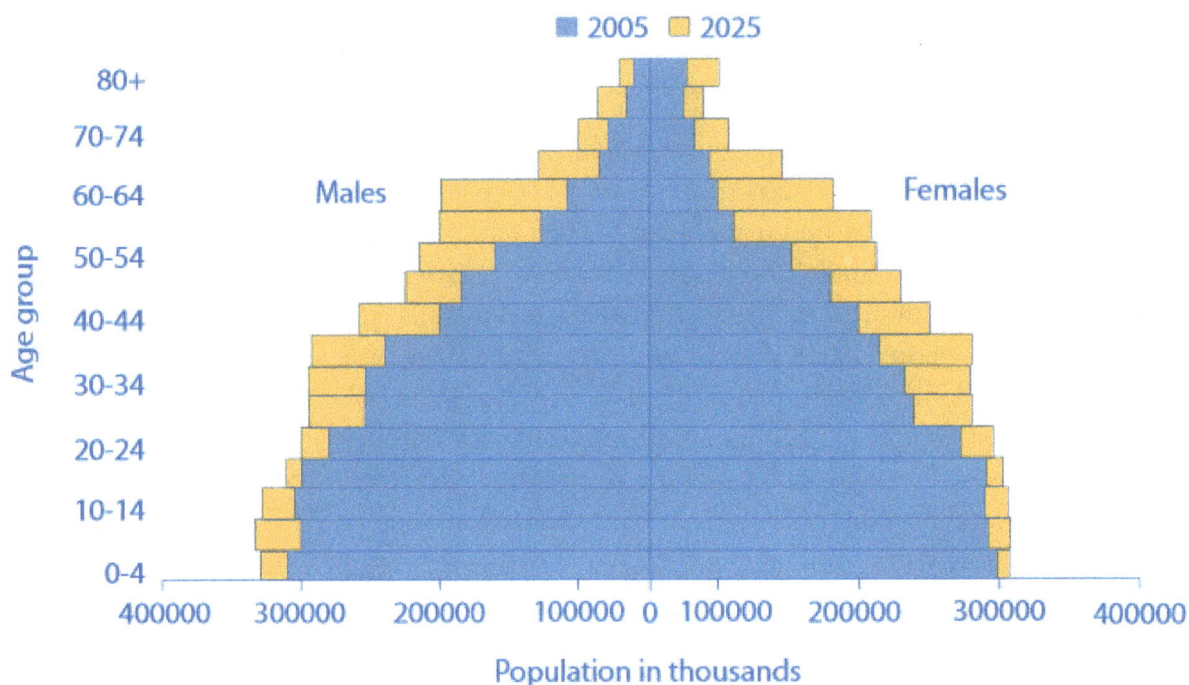

Figure 2. Global population pyramid in 2005 and 2025 [15,25].

The prevention of falls is a considerable challenge for the ageing population. The number of falls increase in magnitude as the number of aged people increase in many populations throughout the world [15]. Falls increase with age because of biological change. Consequently, the number of people aged 80 years and over will trigger a substantial increase of falls and injuries at an anxious rate. Actually, incidence of fall injuries have increased by 131% in the last three decades. The number of injuries caused by falls is predicted to be 100% higher in the year 2030 [15,21].

This applies to developing countries where ageing population is rapidly occurring and where close to 70% of the elderly population lives. To add, "the developed world that became richer before getting older, developing countries are getting older before becoming richer" [26].

The Ontorio working group linked the cause of the high incidence of falls to extrinsic and intrinsic risk factors. The intrinsic risk factors are the physical characteristics, demographics, and general health status of elders; e.g. psychosocial-demographic risks, medical risks and considered as risk and degree of dependency with activity levels. While the extrinsic factors are thought to be related to the physical and socio-economic environment; e.g. balance, slip hazards and vision hazard. [27].

Most falls result from a person's environment. The causes are, especially, the predisposing and precipitating factors of the person's environment. In most studies, about 25 to 45 percent of falls occur because of environmental hazards [28]. The other common causes are gait disturbance and muscle weakness. The risk factors of falls are dizziness, vertigo, drop attacks, postural hypotension, visual impairment, and syncope in patients. Lower extremity muscle weakness is a significant risk factor for falls because it increases the odds of falling fourfold. The other risk factors of falls are having fall history and gait or balance deficits which increases the risk threefold. Other high-risk situations for falls are the use of an assistive device, visual deficit, arthritis, impaired activities of daily living, depression, cognitive impairment, and age over 80 years. Studies reported that, medication increases the risk of falls, especially the use of four or more medications, which have been strongly associated with an increased risk of falls. In particular, the use of psychotropic medications, cardiac drugs including class 1A antiarrhythmic agents, digoxin, diuretics, and anticonvulsants have been implicated in increasing the risk of falls [29,30]. In a social perspective, falls are one of the most common geriatric syndromes because of the threat to the independence of older persons. Between 30 to 40 percent of community-dwelling adults older than 65 years fall each year, and the rates are higher for nursing home residents. Falls are associated with increased morbidity, mortality, and nursing home placement [31,32]. The other risk factors of falls are arthritis, depression and activities of daily living [33,34].

Falling due to fractures is very common in the geriatric population. In Canada, it is stated that a large 23,631 people 59 years and older were hospitalized due to femoral neck fractures. The most frequent cause of hospitalization for 65 years old and older is hip fracture. Femoral neck fractures with dependence in daily activities in patients older than 85 years also increases [35-40].

The American Academy of Family Practice offers a clinical assessment to determine the risk of fractures in the elderly. The risk groups are defined as the conditions shown in Table 1 below.

Clinical Assessments and Interventions for Elderly at Risk for Falls*	
Assessment and risk factor	*Interventions*
Circumstances of previous falls	Changes in environment and activity to reduce the likelihood of recurrent falls
Medication use High-risk medications Four or more medications	Review and reduction of medications
Vision Acuity < 20/60 Decreased depth perception Decreased contrast sensitivity Cataracts	Ample lighting without glare; avoidance of multifocal glasses while walking; referral to an ophthalmologist
Postural blood pressure; ≥ 20 mm Hg drop in systolic pressure, with or without symptoms, repeat immediately or after two minutes of standing	Diagnosis and treatment of underlying cause, if possible; review and reduction of medications; modification of salt restriction; adequate hydration; compensatory strategies; pressure stockings; pharmacologic therapy if the above strategies fail
Balance and gait Patient's report or observation of unsteadiness Impairment on brief assessment	Diagnosis and treatment of underlying cause, if possible; reduction of medications that impair balance; environmental interventions; referral to physical therapist for assistive devices and for gait and progressive balance training
Targeted neurologic examination Impaired proprioception Impaired cognition Decreased muscle strength	Diagnosis and treatment of underlying cause, if possible; increase in proprioceptive input; reduction of medications that impede cognition; awareness on the part of caregivers of cognitive deficits; reduction of environmental risk factors; referral to physical therapist for gait, balance, and strength training
Targeted musculoskeletal examination: examination of legs and feet	Diagnosis and treatment of underlying cause, if possible; referral to physical therapist for strength, range-of-motion, and gait and balance training and for assistive devices; use of appropriate footwear; referral to podiatrist
Targeted cardiovascular examination Syncope Arrhythmia	Referral to cardiologist; carotid-sinus massage
Home hazard evaluation after hospital discharge	Removal of loose rugs and use of night lights, non-slip bath mats, and stair rails; other interventions as necessary

Table 1. Clinical Assessments and Interventions for Older Persons at Risk for Falls

Tinetti ME. Clinical practice. Preventing falls in elderly persons. N Engl J Med 2003;348:45.

Health care services has provided the necessary preventive measures for fall-related fractures in the geriatric population. There are some precautions, in terms of extrinsic factors, that are also needed to be taken to prevent falls. In this regard, the US Preventive Task Force (USPSTF) offers suggestions to prevent fractures in elderly patients [41]. The USPSTF recommendations are given in Table 2 below.

Strength of Recommendations*	
Key clinic Recommendations	Label
Home hazard assessment and modification is recommended for patients with a history of falls.	A
Exercise and physical therapy are recommended to prevent falls and injury from falls.	A
Patients should receive a multifactorial risk assessment and intervention because it is the most consistently effective strategy to prevent falls.	A
Evaluation of medications and withdrawal of medications that increase the risk of falling is recommended.	B
Dual-chamber pacemaker placement is recommended for selected patients with carotid sinus syndrome and syncope.	B
Hip protectors are recommended for patients at high risk of falling in an institutional setting.	B
Patients with a history of falls or with risk factors for falling should undergo a formal evaluation.	C

* U.S. Preventive Services Task Force. Guide to clinical preventive services

Table 2. Recommendations and labels for preventing elderly people from falls

One of the most significant pathology in the geriatric age group is also dementia. The most common cause of dementia in the USA is Alzheimer's disease that has an annual health spending of 192 billion dollars. The cost for health expenditure has been based from a study but the social impact cannot be calculated [41].

4. Dementia in the aged population

The biggest problem is defined as dementia in the aged population. Dementia prevalence is estimated to amount to 24 million and predicted to quadruple by the year 2050 [41]. Dementia is defined as an overall term for diseases and conditions characterized by a decline in memory or other thinking skills that affects a person's ability to perform everyday activities. According to the DSM V criteria, dementia is defined in terms of major and mild neurocognitive disorders. In the epidemiological data, 24.2 million people lived with dementia at that time, with 4.6 million new cases arising every year [3]. In Canada; 2.0% of the population were diagnosed with dementia [11]. Dementia, increases with age, especially over the age of 65 years where it has been often seen by 1.5 times more.

Previous definitions of dementia have often included the requirement of a progressive and irreversible impairment. Dementia related so many things and can occur before or after the age of 65 [42].

Alzheimer's disease (AD) has been one of the top reasons of the dementia which estimates 60-80%. The etiology of Alzheimer's disease shows many reasons, although the exact etiologic factor could not be determined. The early-onset AD is referred to the existence of genetic factors associated with the etiology of APOE. While with the late onset AD, the etiological factors could not be determined [4].

5. Alzheimer's disease epidemiology

Alzheimer's disease is defined as a progressive loss of cognitive function. This function loss history starts with the loss of memory and function, and eventually to all the intellectual activities of daily living, and leads to processes that causes premature death. Beta-amyloid plaques, neurofibrillary tangles, and neurodegeneration are the hallmark pathologic characteristics of AD [4]. In fact, since 20 years ago, there were already initial steps to establish the diagnosis of AD with the onset of symptoms. Etiology has not been fully clarified, but the underlying causes are genetics, age, family history, the Apolipoprotein E-ε4 gene (APOE-ε4), mild cognitive impairment, education level, traumatic brain injury, and cardiovascular risk factors [5].

The prevalence of Alzheimer's disease, according to the countries' health-related database information from Holland, France, Italy, England and USA, is estimated at 3-7% [43].

Memory loss is the most pronounced behavioural abnormality, and is usually the first symptom in Alzheimer's disease. Memory is impaired for recent events, with relative preservation of remote memory. In the early stages of the disease, memory impairment may be an isolated dysfunction, followed in time by the development of impairments of attention, language function (defective word finding with otherwise fluent speech), visuospatial abilities (drawing, route finding), praxis (purposeful movements), calculations, visual, auditory and olfactory perception, problem-solving ability, and judgement. Patients with Alzheimer's disease have difficulty shifting their mental set from one task to another. Depression, personality changes, apathy, and irritability are also common features of the disease. Language abilities and social skills may be remarkably preserved, even in the later stages, and patients with well-established dementia may be able to maintain polite conversations with remarkable skill and thus appear to be intact to the casual observer. Paranoid delusions, illusions, and hallucinations are seen in a minority of patients, usually in the later stages. Up to half of the patients with Alzheimer's disease have limited awareness of their behavioural deficits. It should be emphasized that the behavioural features of this disease are highly variable from patient to patient: some patients may have preserved language function with impaired visuospatial abilities, while other patients at a similar stage in the overall disease process may show the reverse pattern of deficits. Motor function and urinary continence are usually not affected until later. This variability, or heterogeneity, in the behavioural manifestations of the disease is due to variations in the distribution of disease severity in brain regions. For example, patients with severe involvement of the left temporal and parietal cortex will have relatively more marked language dysfunction. The disease is progressive, with survival rates after an onset of 5 to 12 years duration [42,43].

As the elderly population in developed countries increases, it also can not be prevented to have an increase in the prevalence of Alzheimer's disease. This is due to the change in the direction of health policies. The unknown cause and limited treatment cause higher health expenditures and quite large losses in every perspective.

Alzheimer's Disease, has two types of progressive diseases. If the AD starts before 65 years of age, it is defined as early clinical onset. If it starts after 65 years of age, it is defined as late onset AD. Early-onset AD starts in middle age and is implicated in the etiology of genetic predisposition. Late-onset AD is the most commonly seen in the 70-80 age range, and after 65 years, there is a 2-fold increased risk of AD.

Some factors considered to be the etiology of Alzheimer's disease: age, genetics, family history, the Apolipoprotein E-ε4 gene (APOE-ε4), mild cognitive impairment, education level, traumatic brain injury, and cardiovascular risk factors.

Age: Age is associated with the increase in the prevalence of AD. After 65 years of age, it is known that a 2-fold increase likelihood of AD occurs every 5 years. When a person isover 85 years of age, the increased risk becomes 16-fold.

Genetics: There are many studies on this subject. There are some genes and polymorphisms that are genetically determined. These genes and polymorphisms are associated with the pathophysiology of white plaque in AD. Alzheimer's disease pathology in the brain is characterised by the presence of plaques of amyloid β peptides and intraneuronal tangles of hyperphosphorylated forms of microtubule-associated protein tau (MAPT) [44]. It is stated that in the studies of both componentscarry genetic forms of AD. Casual mutations in three genes have been identified in early-onset forms, establishing the central role of amyloid in Alzheimer's disease, which has become to be the most widely studied pathway since these discoveries [45-49]. Twin studies have observed that the transition rate is 80% [50].

In the absence of transitions in all AD patients with the same genes, it has been suggested that the environmental factors are related in the development of the disease. It has been genetically implicated, especially in the early onset of Alzheimer's disease with APOE ε4 allele presence. At the molecular level, especially in transition, Mendelian APP, PSEN1, and PSEN2 mutations were studied [45-49].

Mutations in PSEN1 and PSEN2 are also directly related to amyloid production; they impair the γ-secretase-mediated cleavage of APP, resulting in an increased ratio of amyloid β to amyloid β [51].

The results of the studies that show autosomal dominant Mendelian characteristics found that some genes were involved in the pathology of AD. The late-onset AD is also guilty of the changes in these genes. The genome-wide association and replication of these genes, additionally, have been reported for single nucleotide polymorphisms in or near CR1, PICALM, and BIN1[52]. Continued concerted efforts identified the association with single nucleotide polymorphisms especially in MS4A cluster, CD2AP, CD33, EPHA1, and ABCA7 [52-56].

Apolipoprotein-ε4 (APOE ε4)

Apolipoprotein-ε4 allele is the best known factor for the late-onset and early-onset forms. The Alzheimer's disease risk is increased with having one ε4 allele roughly three-times and those with two ε4 alleles have a roughly 15-times-increased risk, compared with the most common genotype, APOE ε3ε3 [57].

Results of early studies suggested that this risk was greatest in patients who were 60–79 years of age at the onset, a notion confirmed by a study of more than 17,000 individuals with whom the risk of disease in APOE ε4ε4 carriers aged 60–69 years was as much as 35 times higher than that noted in APOE ε3ε3 carriers [58]. In APOE ε4 carriers, the lifetime risk of Alzheimer's disease (an estimate independent of APOE ε3ε3 and the actual probability of developing disease between birth and a given age) at age 85 years was estimated to be as high as 35% for female APOE ε3ε4 carriers and 68% for female APOE ε4ε4 carriers [59].

5.1. Cerebrovascular diseases

Hemorrhagic infarcts, vasculopathy or something which causes changes in white matter cause AD, however, the specific name for this cause or reason has not yet been identified. Infarcts can lead to losses in areas related to memory or due inflammation that occurs in AD [62,63].

5.2. Hypertension

In studies, the hypertension that especially occurs in middle aged people, could cause the onset AD. In many studies, vascular resistance of the resulting protein will lead to the extravasation of the blood-brain barrier and, thus, lead to damage in the cell structure, apoptosis, and damage in the brain. In addition, this may be considered as a cause of AD [62,63].

5.3. Type 2 Diabetes Mellitus

Type 2 DM is accused to be the cause of hyperinsulinemia in AD patients. Ensuring that the peripheral hyperinsulinemia down-regulates the insulin receptors in the brain, under physiological insulin needs provides a transition to the brain and leads to an increase in the IDE found mediated amyloid production [64,65].

5.4. Lipid disorders

Many studies considered cognitive impairment and AD are caused by lipid disorders, although there is no evidence to reveal exactly why. The reason for this is that genetics predisposition and apolipoprotein E, apolipoprotein J (APOJ, CLU), ATP-binding cassette subfamily A member 7 (ABCA7), and sortilin-related receptor (SORL1) are responsible etiology of AD and lipid metabolism [66-68].

5.5. Head injury

In the meta-analysis, it is particularly prevalent in people who underwent a traumatic brain injury with dementia [69-71]. Especially the men are more affected than the women. However, there are inconsistent evidences for head injuries increasing the risk of AD.

6. Alzheimer disease and risk of falls

The prevalence of falls in patients with mild to moderate dementia is at 42% [44]. Cognitive destruction of dementia patients have a worse prognosis than when they fall. In studies, falls are more frequently seen in patients with AD [45]. In the world, the geriatric age population is increasing and consequently the number of patients with AD is also increasing too meaning falls happen in the people in this group, which is a serious problem [44-47].

According to the CDC, every year people aged 65 and over fall [48-49]. Falls can cause fatal and nonfatal injuries, and can increase the risk of early death [50]. In fact, we know that falls are a preventable public health problem, especially for aging communities. In aging societies, Alzheimer diseases is another serious health problem, which is largely seen in developed countries. The death and injury rates that result from falls among older men and women have risen sharply over the past decade (Table 3). Aged people with Alzheimer's Disease are at a particularly high risk of falling. Problems with vision, perception, and balance increase as the Alzheimer's Disease advances, making the risk of a fall more likely [51].

Deaths
In 2011, about 22,900 older adults died from unintentional fall injuries.
Men are more likely than women to die from a fall. After taking age into account, the fall death rate in 2011 was 41% higher for men than for women.
Older whites are 2.7 times more likely to die from falls as their black counterparts.
Rates also differ by ethnicity. Older non-Hispanics have higher fatal fall rates than Hispanics.
Injuries
People age 75 and older who fall are four to five times more likely to be admitted to a long-term care facility for a year or longer, than those age 65 to 74.
Rates of fall-related fractures among older women are more than twice than those for men.
Over 95% of hip fractures are caused by falls. In 2010, there were 258,000 hip fractures and the rate for women was almost twice the rate for men (15).
White women have significantly higher hip fracture rates than black women.

*Centers for Disease Control and Prevention, the National Center for Injury Prevention and Control.

Table 3. Fall-related deaths and injuries*

The annual incidence of Alzheimer's disease patients that experience a fall in their age group is 60-80% of non-AD. Also AD patients are 3 times more likely to carry the risk of fall-related developments fraction [52-55].

Although not proven, there are already studies about the increasing frequency of falls in patients by De Groot et al., [9] and Maruyama et al., [10] that cerebral white matter lesions may relate to cognition and postural balance.

There is not known relation between falls and AD. But, changes in motor movements are thought to be related to the recently impaired cognitive function. It is not known whether changes in motor movement, or cognitive loss in AD and mild cognitive impairment had previously occurred [46-57]. Stark SL et al., [58] considered that motor movements are affected before than the cognitive impairment and is argued that the increase of brain amyloid levels increase the risk of falling.

Ogama N et al., [59] declared that AD patients with falls have higher white matter lesions (WML) than patients without falls. The posture and gait performance of the AD patients with falls were lower than patients without falls. It has been found that, the periventricular hyperintensity in frontal caps and occipital WMLs were strong predictors for falls, even after potential risk factors were considered. About the risk of dementia and AD patients, regional WMLs visualisation by the the brain magnetic resonance may greatly help to diagnose dementia in the elderly with a higher risk of falls. Regional white matter burden, independent of cognitive decline, correlates with balance/gait disturbance and predicts falls in elderly with aMCI and AD [59].

In dementia, many risk factors were studied. The most common risk factors for falls in patients with AD that are related to cognitive impairment and dementia are: gait and balance disturbances, behavioral disorders, visual problems, malnutrition, adverse effects of drugs, fear of falling, neurocardiovascular instability (particularly orthostatic hypotension), and environmental hazards.

Based on data from studies, a multifaceted intervention, including a physical exercise programme, and a modification of the risk factors may prevent falls in older people with cognitive impairment and dementia. Lorbach ER et al., considered [60] that age, history of falls, motor impairment, visual disturbance, cognitive disfunction, behavioral disturbance, side effects of prescription drugs, and the presence of risky behaviors are risk factors of falls. NutriAlz' study declared that the risk of falls are related with the history of falls, nutritional status and arthritis [61]. Walking is an automatic process until it is necessary to deviate from the learned program. Most of the locomotion involves intention and therefore, there are cognitive inputs of various degrees.

In AD and the other dementia diseases, cognitive impairment will have a negative effect on all aspects of gait performance and progressive decline in cognition. This may cause a concomitant disorganization of the network that controls locomotion, leading to an impaired gait timing and postural control.

A disintegration of a higher cortical sensory function and a particularly involving perceptual-motor integration may represent in AD patients. Because of this disintegration of the various components, previously learned routine motor functions "breaks down" due to visuo-spatial integration and other functions of higher cortical perception, an unconscious component in the network of motor control. In AD patients, both constructional and ideomotor apraxia at all stages of the disease occur. Alternatively, as a result of trying to compensate for an impaired higher cortical sensory integration and competition for attentional resources, the control of timing in the cerebellum executes programs with variable output, leading to the variability of stepping during the stride with subsequent gait unsteadiness and ultimately leads to falling [62].

Dementia and AD with frontal cognitive impairment is reported to cause deterioration of walking in patients [63]. In the study Coelho et al., [64] AD's mild/moderate stages indicate that the difference between the kinematic parameters is walking. Moderate stages of AD patients had shorter stride lengths and walked more slowly than patients who were in the mild stage. In the study of Maggio et al., [65] the caregivers are the risk factor of AD because of caregiver stress.

7. Other risk factors of falls in Alzheimer disease

Physiological and cognitive changes and other functional disabilities occur in patients with AD. The experimental or epidemiological studies show that there is more than one etiologic factor that may be responsible for the risk of falls.

Age: Age is seen as the most important etiologic factor. Both AD prevalence and falls increase with ageing. In Nutrialz study, the prevalence increase by 10% with ageing and is increases every 5 years [61]. It is known that, with ageing, dementia, AD, and falls increase. The loss of abilities is related to ageing.

Education level: In the study of Ott et al., [66] high education level is stated to be related to AD. It was especially noted that increased levels of education delay the onset of AD. With a higher education level, neural reserve and neural network capacities are higher, and this delayed the neurodegeneration [67,68]. The effects of education, job and entertainment experiences lead to the efficiency of neural reserves.

Functional Ability and Falls: Normal ageing involves vision, hearing, vestibular, and somatosensory changes in the primary sensory areas. Thus, a more cognitive effort may be required to accommodate these systemic changes. The progressive decline in cognitive functions may lead to the disorganization of the network that controls locomotion, leading to impaired gait speed, timing, and poor postural control [70].

Recent Falling History: The risk of falls is increasing with AD patients that have a previous falling history. This is influenced by, because of recent experiences, fear of falling. Fear of falling are influenced by spatial and temporal parameters [71-72]. In this subject, there are many evidences. Especially, the history of falling is the main risk factor in elderly people and in patients with AD.

Gait: In AD patients, stride length variability at all walking speeds may contribute to the increased incidence of falls [73].

Global Brain Atrophy: White matter lesions in older adults are also associated with gait and balance impairment, cognitive impairment, and frequent falling. Yamaha et al., [74]. stated that patients with cognitive disorders, global brain atrophy is an independent factor for falling in AD patients.

Medication: In AD patients, one of the risk factors for falls is the medication. In the study of Epstein et al., [75] the medication increases the falls. Even after the medication has been changed, medication side effects are still thought to be the cause of the vast majority of falls.

7.1. Preventing falls

Older adults can keep on their independence for their daily life activities and reduce their experience of falling through exercising regularly, asking their doctor to revise their medicine use due to dizziness, having their eyes checked, and making their homes safer [50,77,78].

Because half of all falls occur at home, below are some suggested steps that may be considered to make the home safer (Table 4) [51,79].

Remove things you can trip over, such as papers, books, clothes, and shoes, from stairs and places where you walk.
Remove small throw rugs or use double-sided tape to keep the rugs from slipping.
Keep the items you use often in cabinets you can reach easily without using a step stool.
Have grab bars put next to your toilet and in the tub or shower.
Use non-slip mats in the bathtub and on shower floors.
Improve the lighting in your home. As you get older, you need brighter lights to see well. Lamp shades or frosted bulbs can reduce glare.
Put handrails and lights in all staircases.
Wear shoes that give good support and have thin non-slip soles. Avoid wearing slippers and athletic shoes with deep treads.

Table 4. Safety tips for preventing falls at home

Fall prevention for people with Alzheimer's Disease and other types of dementia is vital. The key point for reducing falls in people with dementia is to understand why they fall and what causes the falls (Figure 3) [78]. Restlessness, discomfort or pain, hunger or thirst, a need to use the bathroom, boredom, and loneliness were other contributors to falls [78-81].

Some studies indicate that cognitive impairment is associated with Alzheimer disease and increase fall risk among older adults. Strategies including multifactorial assessment should be considered to prevent the risk of falling [24,25,82]. Falls are a prevalent health problem in the geriatric population and can result in severe somatic and psychological consequences. Fall risk assessment can provide knowledge to make and develop suitable interventions for identifing persons at risk [21,83].

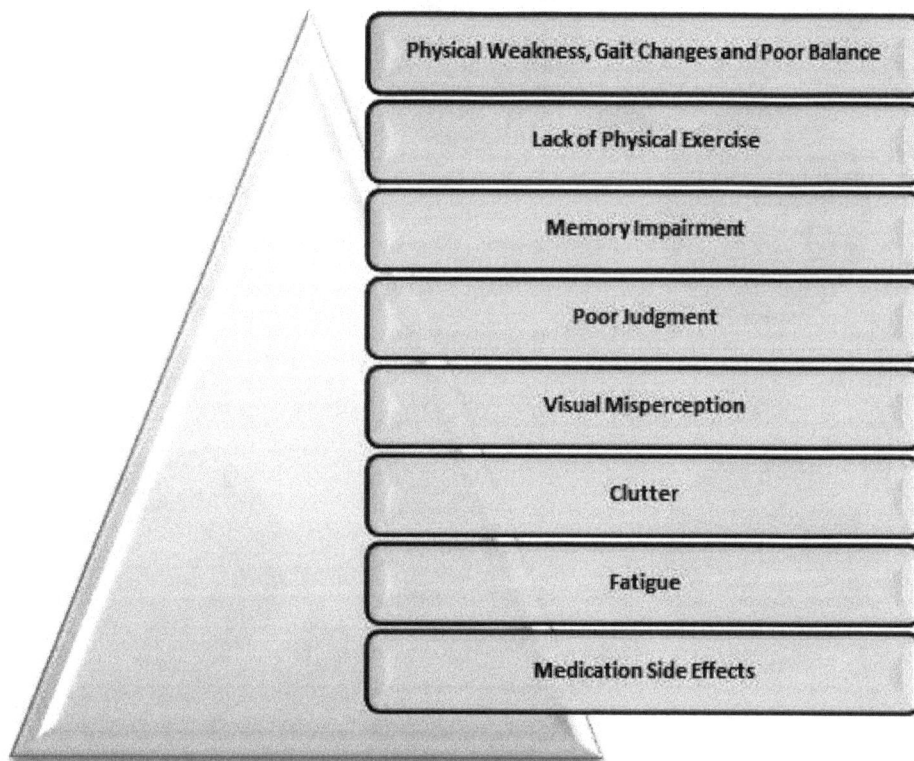

Figure 3. Causes of Falls among People with Alzheimer's Disease

8. How can we avoid accidents and reduce the risk of falls?

Aged people with dementia want to carry on their everyday life at home for as long as possible. However, it can be difficult managing everyday situations if you have dementia, particularly as the dementia progresses and as you get older. In conclusion, some people may not be as safe at home as they used to be. Some risk factors and suggested ways to manage them were mentioned below [84].

Occupational therapy provides practical support to help people do their day-to-day tasks, hobbies, interests, and activities (Figure 4 and 5). People who want to take an occupational therapy assessment can consult their local social services or their psychology experts related to occupational therapy [84].

Other preventions to reduce the risk of falls are: store dangerous substances safely, improve home environment, manage daily activities such as cooking or bathing through adaptations, avoid fire including fitting smoke alarms and carbon monoxide detectors, stay safe outdoors, use support networks, arrange access especially for family member or care worker, and record contact names and numbers belong to carers, friends, or family members [84].

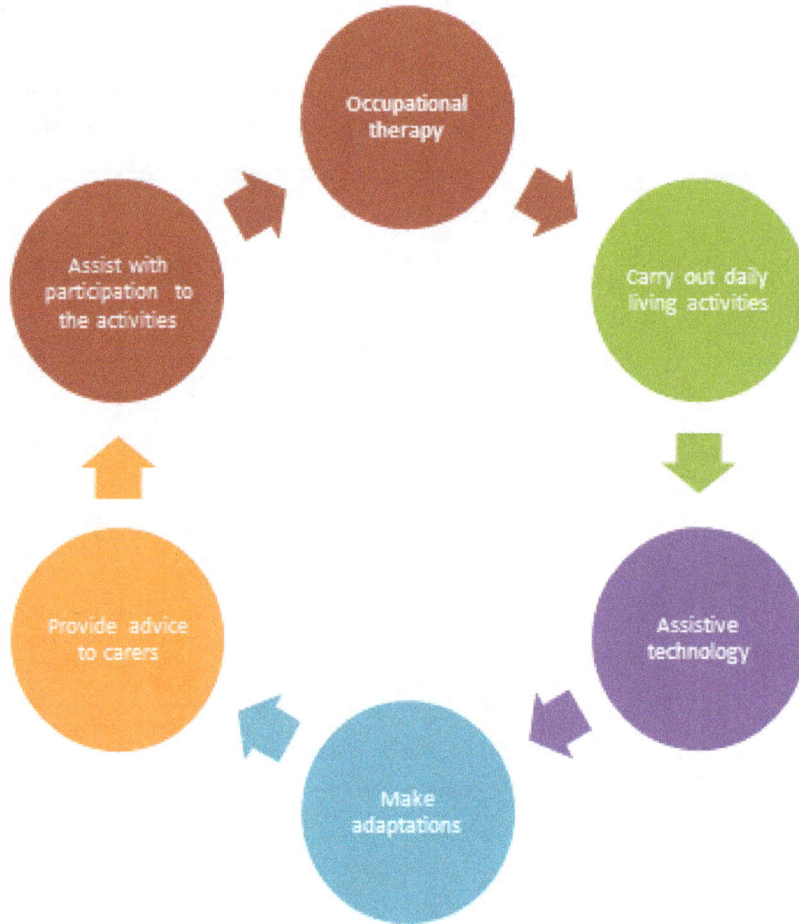

Figure 4. Seek advice from an occupational therapist.

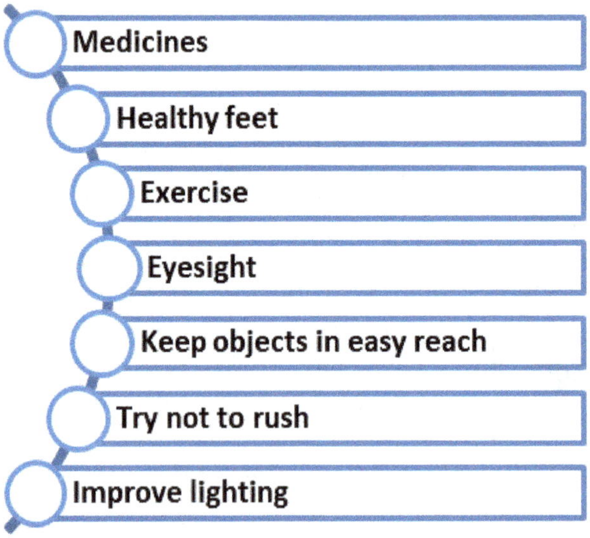

Figure 5. Steps to reduce the risk of falling at home.

9. Conclusion

With ageing, the risk of dementia and falls prevalence increases. Falls are one of the important risks for comorbidity and mortality in the aged population. Preventing strategies must be performed and must be related with the individual as well as the health services and the politics area. Only the implementation of prevention services may be solve this problem because the dementia and AD have a progressive decline process and there is currently no known alternative treatment for these pathologic conditions.

Author details

Aysegul Uludag*, Sibel Cevizci and Ahmet Uludag

*Address all correspondence to: draysegululudag@gmail.com

Canakkale Onsekiz Mart University, Faculty of Medicine, Department of Family Medicine, Canakkale, Turkey

References

[1] Birren JE. The Psycology of Aging, Prentice Hall, Inc. New Jersey; 1982.

[2] Freedman VA, Martin LG, Schoeni RF. Recent trends in disability and functioning among older adults in the United States: a systematic review. JAMA 2002;288(24) 3137-46.

[3] Ferri CP, Prince M, Brayne C, Brodaty H, Fratiglioni L, Ganguli M, Hall K, Hasegawa K, Hendrie H, Huang Y et al. Alzheimer's Disease International. Global prevalence of dementia: a Delphi consensus study. Lancet 2005 17;366(9503) 2112-7.

[4] Thies W, Bleiler L. Alzheimer's disease facts and figures. Alzheimer's Dementia 2013;9(2) 208–45.

[5] Serrano-Pozo A, Frosch MP, Masliah E, Hyman BT. Neuropathological alterations in Alzheimer disease. Cold Spring Harb Perspect Med. 2011;1(1) 24-30.

[6] Morris JC, Rubin EH, Morris EJ, Mandel SA. Senile dementia of the Alzheimer's type: An important risk factor for serious falls. J Gerontol 1987;42 412–17.

[7] Tchalla AE, Lachal F, Cardinaud N, Saulnier I, Rialle V, Preux PM, Dantoine T. Preventing and managing indoor falls with home-based technologies in mild and moderate Alzheimer's disease patients: pilot study in a community dwelling. Dement Geriatr Cogn Disord. 2013;36(3-4) 251-61.

[8] http://www.mayoclinic.org/diseases-conditions/alzheimers-disease/basics/complications/con-20023871 (Accesed date August, 23,2014)

[9] De Groot JC, De Leeuw FE, Oudkerk M, et al. Cerebral white matter lesions and cognitive function: The Rotterdam scan study. Ann Neurol 2000;47 145–51.

[10] Maruyama M, Matsui T, Tanji H, et al. Cerebrospinal fluid tau protein and periventricular white matter lesions in patients with mild cognitive impairment: Implications for two major pathways. Arch Neurol 2004; 61 716–20.

[11] Turcotte M, Schellenberg G. A portrait of seniors in Canada [Internet]. Ottawa: Statistics Canada; 2006. http://www.statcan.gc.ca/pub/89-519-x/89-519-x2006001-eng.pdf (Accesed date August, 23,2014)

[12] Park CR. Cognitive effects of insulin in the central nervous system. Neurosci Biobehav Rev 2001;25(4) 311–23.

[13] Masud T, Morris RO. Epidemiology of falls. Age Ageing 2001;30(suppl 4) 3-7.

[14] Tinetti ME. Factors associated with serious injury during falls by ambulatory nursing home residents. Journal of the American Geriatrics Society 1987;35 644-48.

[15] WHO Global Report on Falls Prevention in Older Age. WHO 2007.

[16] Liang W, Liu Y, Weng X. An epidemiological study on injury of the community-dwelling elderly in Beijing. Chinese Journal of Disease Control and Prevention 2004; 8(6) 489-92.

[17] Yoshida H, Kim H. Frequency of falls and their prevention (in Japanese). Clinical Calcium 2006; 16(9) 1444-50.

[18] Rubenstein LZ. Falls in older people:epidemiology, risk factors and strategies for prevention. Age Ageing 2006;35 32-40.

[19] Stevens JA et al. Fatalities and Injuries From Falls Among Older Adults, United States, 1993-2003 and 2001-2005. Journal of the American Medical Association 2007; 297(1) 32-3.

[20] Division of Aging and Seniors, PHAC. Canada Report on senior's fall in Canada. Ontario, Division of Aging and Seniors. Public Health Agency of Canada 2005.

[21] Kannus P et al. Fall-induced deaths among elderly people. American Public Health Association 2005;95(3) 422-24.

[22] National Council on Ageing. Falls among older adults: risk factors and prevention strategies. In Fall free: promoting a national falls prevention action plan. J.A. Stevens Eds, 2005.

[23] Hernandez JL et al. Trend in hip fracture epidemiology over a 14-year period in a Spanish population. Osteoporosis International, 2006;17 464-70.

[24] World Health Organization. Active Ageing: A Policy Framework. Geneva 2002.

[25] United Nations (UN). World Population Prospects: The 2004 Revision. New York, USA.

[26] Tromp AM, Pluijm SMF, Smit JH, et al. Fall-risk screening test: a prospective study on predictors for falls in community-dwelling elderly. J Clin Epidemiol 2001;54(8) 837–44.

[27] Prevention of Falls and Fall-Related Injuries – Ontario Health Technology Assessment Series 2008;8 (2).

[28] Tinetti ME, Speechley M, Ginter SF. Risk factors for falls among elderly persons living in the community. N Engl J Med 1988;319 1701-7.

[29] Rubenstein LZ, Josephson KR. The epidemiology of falls and syncope. Clin Geriatr Med 2002;18 141-58.

[30] Centers for Disease Control and Prevention. Falls among older adults: summary of research findings. Accessed online January 26, 2005, at: http://www.cdc.gov/ncipc/pub-res/toolkit/SummaryOfFalls.htm

[31] Tinetti ME. Clinical practice. Preventing falls in elderly persons. N Engl J Med 2003;348:42-9.

[32] Nevitt MC, Cummings SR, Kidd S, Black D. Risk factors for recurrent nonsyncopal falls. A prospective study. JAMA 1989;261 2663-8.

[33] American Geriatrics Society, British Geriatrics Society, and American Academy of Orthopaedic Surgeons Panel on Falls Prevention. Guideline for the prevention of falls in older persons. J Am Geriatr Soc 2001;49 664-72.

[34] Leipzig RM, Cumming RG, Tinetti ME. Drugs and falls in older people: a systematic review and meta-analysis: II. Cardiac and analgesic drugs. J Am Geriatr Soc 1999;47 40-50.

[35] Leipzig RM, Cumming RG, Tinetti ME. Drugs and falls in older people: a systematic review and meta-analysis: I. Psychotropic drugs. J Am Geriatr Soc 1999;47:30-9.

[36] Rao SS. Prevention of Falls in Older Patients Am Fam Physician 2005;72 (81) 93-4.

[37] Papadimitropoulos EA, Coyte PC, Josse RG, et al. Current and projected rates of hip fracture in Canada. CMAJ. 1997;157(10) 1357–63.

[38] Canadian Community Health Survey. Detailed information for 2003.

[39] Peel NM, Kassulke DJ, McClure RJ. Population based study of hospi talised fall related injuries in older people. Inj Prev. 2002;8(4) 280–3.

[40] Maravic M, Le Bihan C, Landais P, et al. Incidence and cost of osteoporotic fractures in France during 2001. A methodological approach by the national hospital database. Osteoporos Int. 2005;16(12) 1475–80.

[41] U.S. Preventive Services Task Force. Guide to clinical preventive services: report of the U.S. Preventive Services Task Force. 2d ed. Baltimore: Williams & Wilkins, 1996.

[42] Robert P, Wilcock FKG. Dementia. J. Grimely Evans, T. Franklin Williams (Ed). Oxford Medical Publications, 2nd Edition. Oxford University Press, 2002.

[43] Takizawa C, Thompson PL, Van Walsem A, Faure C, Maier WC. Epidemiological and Economic Burden of Alzheimer's Disease: A Systematic Literature Review of Data across Europe and the United States of America J Alzheimer's Dis. 2014 26. [Epub ahead of print].

[44] Plassman BL, Havlik RJ, Steffens DC, Helms MJ, Newman TN, Drosdick D, et al. Documented head injury in early adulthood and risk of Alzheimer's disease and other dementias. Neurology 2000;55(8) 1158–66.

[45] Horikawa E, Matsui T, Arai H, et al. Risk of falls in Alzheimer's disease: a prospective study. Int Med. 2005;44:717–21.

[46] Webster KE, Merory JR, Wittwer JE. Gait variability in community dwelling adults with Alzheimer disease. Alzheimer Dis Assoc Disord. 2006;20 37-40.

[47] Glickstein J, Tideiksaar R. Risk of falls and injury in Alzheimer's disease. Focus Geriatr Care Rehabil. 1998;12 2-12.

[48] Chong RK, Horak FB, Frank J, Kaye J. Sensory organization for balance: specific deficits in Alzheimer's but not in Parkinson's disease. J Gerontol A Biol Sci Med Sci. 1999;54:122-28.

[49] CDC. Falls Among Older Adults: An Overview. http://www.cdc.gov/homeandrecreationalsafety/falls/adultfalls.html (Accessed August 15, 2013).

[50] Centers for Disease Control and Prevention, National Center for Injury Prevention and Control. Web–based Injury Statistics Query and Reporting System (WISQARS) [online]. Accessed August 15, 2013.

[51] Gang L, Sufang JYS. The incidence status on injury of the community-dwelling elderly in Beijing (in Chinese). Chinese Journal of Preventive Medicine, 2006;40(1) 3713.

[52] Gillespie, LD, Robertson, MC, Gillespie, WH, Sherrington C, Gates S, Clemson LM, Lamb SE. Interventions for preventing falls in older people living in the community. Cochrane Database of Systematic Reviews 2012;9.

[53] Olsson RH, Jr, Wambold S, Brock B, Waugh D, Sprague H. Visual spatial abilities and fall risk: an assessment tool for individuals with dementia. J Gerontol Nurs. 2005;31 45-51.

[54] Shaw FE. Falls in cognitive impairment and dementia. Clin Geriatr Med. 2002; 18 159-73.

[55] Sheridan PL, Hausdorff JM. The role of higher-level cognitive function in gait: executive dysfunction contributes to fall risk in Alzheimer's disease. Dement Geriatr Cogn Disord. 2007;24 125-37.

[56] Alexander NB, Hausdorff JM. Guest editorial: linking thinking, walking, and falling. J Gerontol A Biol Sci Med Sci 2008;63 1325–28.

[57] Liu-Ambrose TY, Ashe MC, Graf P, Beattie BL, Khan KM. Increased risk of falling in older community-dwelling women with mild cognitive impairment. Phys Ther 2008; 88 1482–91.

[58] Stark SL, Roe CM, Grant EA, Hollingsworth H, Benzinger TL, Fagan AM, et al. Preclinical Alzheimer disease and risk of Falls Neurology, 2013;82(5) 437-43.

[59] Ogama N, Sakurai T, Shimizu A, Toba K.J. Regional white matter lesions predict falls in patients with amnestic mild cognitive impairment and Alzheimer's disease. Am Med Dir Assoc. 2014;15(1) 36-41.

[60] Lorbach ER, Webster KE, Menz HB, Wittwer JE, Merory JR. Physiological falls risk assessment in older people with Alzheimer's disease. Dement Geriatr Cogn Disord. 2007;24 260-265.

[61] Salva A, Roque´ M, Rojano X, Inzitari M, Andrieu S, Schiffrin EC, Guigoz Y et al. Falls and Risk Factors for Falls in Community-Dwelling Adults With Dementia (NutriAlz Trial) Alzheimer Disease Ass. Disorder. 2012;26(1) 74-80.

[62] Sheridan PL, Hausdorff JM. The role of higher-level cognitive function in gait: executive dysfunction contributes to fall risk in Alzheimer's disease Dement Geriatr Cogn Disord. 2007; 24(2) 125–37.

[63] Holtzer R, Verghese J, Xue X, Lipton RB. Cognitive processes related to gait velocity: Results from the Einstein Aging Study. Neuropsychology 2006; 20 215–23.

[64] De Melo Coelho FG, Stella F, de Andrade LP, Barbieri FA, Galduróz RFS, et al. Gait and risk of falls associated with frontal cognitive functions at different stages of Alzheimer's disease Neuropsychology, Development, and Cognition. Section B, Aging, Neuropsychology and Cognition 2012;19(5) 644-56.

[65] Maggio D, Ercolani S, Andreani S, Ruggiero C, Mariani E, Mangialasche F, et al. Emotional and psychological distress of persons involved in the care of patients with Alzheimer disease predicts falls and fractures in their care recipients. Dement Geriatr Cogn Disord. 2010;30(1) 33-8.

[66] Ott A, Breteler MM, van Harskamp F, et al. Prevalence of Alzheimer's disease and vascular dementia: association with education. The Rotterdam study. BMJ 1995;310 970-3.

[67] Roe CM, Xiong C, Miller JP, Morris JC. Education and Alzheimer disease without dementia: support for the cognitive reserve hypothesis. Neurology 2007;68 223-8.

[68] Bennett DA, Wilson RS, Schneider JA, et al. Education modifies the relation of AD pathology to level of cognitive function in older persons. Neurology. 2003;60 1909-15.

[69] Sheridan PL, Hausdorff JM. The role of higher-level cognitive function in gait: executive dysfunction contributes to fall risk in Alzheimer's disease. Dement Geriatr Cogn Disord. 2007;24 125-37.

[70] Franssen EH, Souren LE, Torossian CL, Reisberg B. Equilibrium and limb coordination in mild cognitive impairment and mild Alzheimer's disease. J Am Geriatr Soc. 1999;47:463-9.

[71] Chamberlin ME, Fulwider BD, Sanders SL, Medeiros JM. Does fear of falling influence spatial and temporal gait parameters in elderly persons beyond changes associated with normal aging? J Gerontol A Biol Sci Med Sci. 2005;60 1163-7.

[72] Nakamura T, Meguro K, Sasaki H. Relationship between falls and stride length variability in senile dementia of the Alzheimer type. Gerontology 1996;42 108-13.

[73] Webster KE, Merory JR, Wittwer JE. Gait Variability in Community Dwelling Adults With Alzheimer Disease Alzheimer Dis Assoc Disord 2006;20 37–40

[74] Yamada M, Takechi H, Mori S, Aoyama T, Arai H. Global brain atrophy is associated with physical performance and the risk of falls in older adults with cognitive impairment Geriatr Gerontol Int 2013; 13 437–42.

[75] Epstein NU, Guo R, Farlow MR, Singh JP, Fisher M. Medication for Alzheimer's disease and associated fall hazard: a retrospective cohort study from the Alzheimer's Disease Neuroimaging Initiative. Drugs Aging. 2014;31(2) 125-9.

[76] Moyer VA. Prevention of Falls in Community-Dwelling Older Adults: U.S. Preventive Services Task Force Recommendation Statement. Annals of Internal Medicine 2012;157(3) 197–204.

[77] Nicole L. Baker, Michael N. Cook, H. Michael Arrighi and Roger Bullock: Hip fracture risk and subsequent mortality among Alzheimer's disease patients in the United Kingdom, 1988–2007 Oxford Textbook of Geriatric Medicine 2010;18.

[78] Heerema E. Causes of Falls in People with Dementia. Understanding Why People Fall Can Help Reduce and Prevent Falls. http://alzheimers.about.com/od/symptomsofalzheimers/a/Causes-of-Falls-in-People-With-Dementia.html (accessed August 13. 2014).

[79] Age and Ageing. Hip fracture risk and subsequent mortality among Alzheimer's disease patients in the United Kingdom, 1988–2007. Accessed September 25, 2012. http://ageing.oxfordjournals.org/content/40/1/49.abstract?sid=02dbc022-d8eb-4fb3-a547-3f781daf1540

[80] Fischer Center for Alzheimer's Research Foundation. People With Alzheimer's at High Risk of Falls and Injury. Accessed September 25, 2012. http://www.alzinfo.org/04/articles/people-alzheimers-high-risk-falls-injury

[81] The Royal Melbourne Hospital. Falls and Dementia. Accessed September 25, 2012. www.mednwh.unimelb.edu.au/vic_falls/pdf_docs/Eric_Seal.

[82] Mignardot JB, Beauchet O, Annweiler C, Cornu C, Deschamps T. Postural sway, falls, and cognitive status: a cross-sectional study among older adults. J Alzheimers Dis. 2014;41(2):431-9.

[83] Kalache A, Keller I (2000). The greying world: a challenge for the 21st century. Science Progress, 83(1):33-54.

[84] Falls. Safety in the home. http://alzheimers.org.uk/site/scripts/documents_info.php?documentID=145 (Accessed September 25, 2012)

4

Recent Progress in the Identification of Non-Invasive Biomarkers to Support the Diagnosis of Alzheimer's Disease in Clinical Practice and to Assist Human Clinical Trials

Francois Bernier, Pavan Kumar, Yoshiaki Sato and
Yoshiya Oda

Additional information is available at the end of the chapter

1. Introduction

Alzheimer's disease (AD) is a neurodegenerative disorder that manifests itself by progressive dementia accompanied by memory deterioration usually in elderlies and is becoming the public health crisis of the 21st century. Currently, there are an estimated 35 Million patients affected by the disease, and this number is expected to burgeon to 115 million by the year 2050 (WHO, 2012). In the United States alone, one patient is diagnosed with AD every 67 seconds according to the Alzheimer's Association website.

This situation is very alarming since Alzheimer's disease has been a graveyard for drug developers with an astonishing 99.6% of trials of potential Alzheimer's treatments aimed at preventing, curing or improving the symptoms of the disease failing or being discontinued from 2002 to 2014 [1]. Although there are FDA approved drugs available including acetylcholine esterase inhibitors (donepezil, rivastigmine, galantamine) and the NMDA receptor antagonist memantine that have been useful in temporarily alleviating short-term memory problems or improving daily functions, they are ineffective in stopping disease progression.

AD is characterized by the presence of amyloid plaques in brain and it is hypothesized that the increase levels of toxic Amyloid beta oligomers and protofibrils leads to Tau neurofibrillary tangles formation, loss of synaptic connections and selective neuronal cell death in the brain (Figure 1) and this sequence of events is referred as the amyloid cascade hypothesis [2]. The amyloid plaques are mostly composed of amyloid-beta peptides (Abeta 40-42) thought to be toxic once they self-aggregate and subsequently bind to a cell surface to disrupt neuronal signaling and cell viability [3]. It is initially thought that downstream to this event is the formation of neurofibrillary tangles composed of hyperphosphorylated Tau protein. Such hyperphosphorylation is an indicator of neuronal cell death in numerous neurodegenerative disorders or brain injuries [4, 5] indicating that both abnormal processes can take place independently [6]. Two key enzymes necessary for the cleavage of the Amyloid Precursor Protein (APP) to generate Amyloid-beta peptides are the gamma and beta-secretase. According to the amyloid cascade, it is thought that developing Inhibitors of those enzymes would prevent amyloid formation and stop disease progression. Several companies have therefore been testing such inhibitors in human trials. Unfortunately, this has proven to be harder than anticipated. While Bace1 inhibitors trials outcomes are not yet known at the time of this writing, gamma-secretase inhibitors had disappointing results in late-stage trials where worsening of cognition was observed [7]. The reason for this is not totally clear, but the fact that gamma-secretase is responsible for the cleavage of multiple substrates including NOTCH protein may have been a contributing factor.

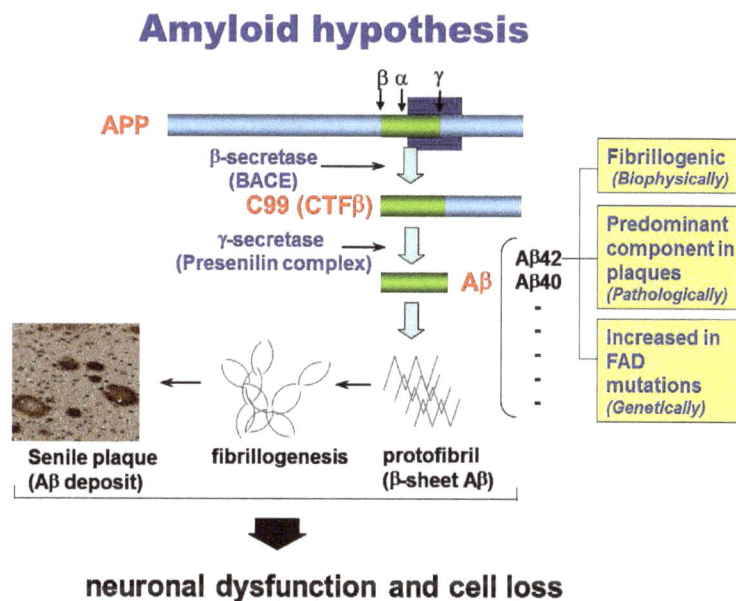

Figure 1. Transmembrane APP protein can be cleaved by three proteases; Beta, Alpha, and Gamma-secretase. Cleavage by B-secretase and G-secretase produces Abeta peptides (mainly 40 and 42). Aggregation of Abeta peptides into toxic oligomers and protofibrils to brain cells is a critical event prior to Abeta plaques formation and disruption of neuronal function and cellular loss.

Other clinical approaches around the amyloid cascade are focusing on passive immunization using administered human monoclonal antibodies against the amyloid-beta peptides, oligomers, protofibrils or plaques [8-10]. Several advanced phase 2 and 3 trials are still ongoing (Table 1) but at least one phase 3 trial outcome, although it did not meet its endpoints has revealed that patients with the mild form of the disease seemed to respond better to treatment [11, 12].

Based on this data, it appears that it might be too late to stop disease progression in patient with mild-to-moderate to severe AD patients with anti-amyloid therapies, so companies are now focusing their efforts on testing those drugs, including beta-secretase inhibitors, in early Mild Cognitive Impairment patients (MCI) which are known to convert to AD more rapidly, especially if patients test positive for amyloid deposition using Positron Emission Tomography scans (PET) [13, 14]. It also comes as no surprise that companies developing these new therapies are now adding being positive on amyloid PET scan as entry criteria in recent clinical trials [15] (table1). Unfortunately, the cost of amyloid PET imaging is very expensive, and PET centers are not currently available worldwide [16-18]. Even if Amyloid-PET is proven to be useful to identify a target patient population, it is important to also develop a non-invasive biomarker that could either be singly used to identify amyloid positive patients or used as a first-line test before Amyloid PET imaging confirmation.

Drug	Trial phase	Patient population	Enriched Study population	Amyloid PET	CSF Abeta	CSF Tau	FDG-PET	VMRI
			Anti-amyloid passive immunotherapies					
Solanezumab	Phase 3	mild AD	yes (Amyloid PET)	yes	yes	yes	no	yes
Gantenerumab	Phase 2/3	autosomal-dominant AD	yes (Amyloid PET)	yes	yes	yes	yes	yes
Crenezumab	Phase 2	mild-moderate AD	no	yes	yes	yes	yes	no
		autosomal-dominant AD	yes (genetics)	yes	no	no	yes	yes
Ban2401	Phase 2	early AD	yes (Amyloid PET)	yes	yes	yes	no	yes
BIIB037	Phase 1	prodromal/mild AD	yes (Amyloid PET)	yes	no	no	no	no
LY3002813	Phase 1	mild-moderate AD	yes (Amyloid PET)	no	no	no	no	no
MEDI1814	Phase 1	mild-moderate AD	no	no	yes	no	no	no
			Bace inhibitors					
MK-8931	Phase 2/3	mild-moderate AD	no	yes	no	no	no	yes
	Phase 3	prodromal AD	yes (Amyloid PET)	yes	no	no	no	yes
E2609	Phase 2	prodromal AD/mild AD	yes (Amyloid PET)	yes	yes	yes	no	no
JNJ-54861911	Phase 1	prodromal AD	yes (Amyloid PET)	yes	yes	no	no	no
AZD3293	Phase 1	mild/moderate AD	no	no	yes	no	no	no

Source: Clinicaltrial.Gov and various press releases.

Table 1. Please add caption

In this book chapter, we will review the recent progress in the development of non-invasive AD biomarkers that could be used for such purpose by various research groups with a focus on AD biomarkers our group recently identified in patients' plasma.

2. The diagnosis of Alzheimer' Disease and the need for non-invasive markers

The disease is difficult to diagnose correctly even with the availability of cognitive tests and sophisticated Imaging technologies that include MRI, FDG-PET and Amyloid PET imaging. Currently, a diagnosis of probable AD is made using NINCDS-ADRDA criteria but this is usually possible when the condition has developed and progressed to a point where neuronal cell death and/or irreparable damages have already occurred [19]. While the accuracy of this test was thought to be around 80-90% when it was developed in the early 80's, it's accuracy, especially to diagnose patients at the early stage of the disease, is much lower which further complicates AD biomarker discovery.

The inability to correctly diagnose AD has also probably negatively affected the development of novel therapies aiming at stopping the amyloid cascade via gamma-secretase inhibitors as well passive immunization therapies using antibodies against abeta peptides or abeta plaques [7, 11]. The possible inclusion of patients suffering from non-AD dementia in those trials may have been a contributing factor to those failures.

As a result, research efforts have intensified exponentially in the recent years to identify and develop biomarkers that could be used for diagnosing AD early to support clinical practice and clinical drug development [20].

Much of these efforts have initially focus on looking at pathological changes of amyloid beta peptides, Abeta 40/42 in CSF as well as P-Tau and T-Tau and has eventually led to the development of a model that define Alzheimer's disease progression [6, 21, 22]. In that original model, gradual reduction in Abeta 42 is observed in CSF, presumably due to the aggregation of the peptide in brain and formation of plaques which is followed by gradual elevation of P-TAU and TAU in CSF, indicators of neuronal cell death or injury[23, 24]. The model was initially received with great interest because it described the temporal evolution of AD biomarkers in relation to each other and the onset and progression of clinical symptoms. However, emerging evidence appeared that challenges this model's assumptions. Refinements to the model now include indexing of individuals by the time rather than clinical symptom severity.; incorporation of inter-individual cognitive impairment variability in relation to AD pathophysiology progression; modifications to when some biomarkers changes sequentially appear; and acknowledgement that the two major proteinopathies in AD, amyloid beta (Abeta) and tau, might be initiated separately from one another in sporadic AD[6].

Although useful to assist clinical diagnosis of AD with enough sensitivity and specificity [23, 25], stiff barriers exist that prevent the comprehensive utilization of those markers by physicians and especially primary care doctors. Lumbar puncture, for example, that is required to collect CSF is still a delicate medical intervention in several developed countries and is also accompanied by increased frequency of headaches [26].The nature of the Amyloid peptides itself is also complicating the picture. Recent data have indeed shown that the Abeta 42 peptides are prone to stick to collection tubes and their detected concentration is affected by various parameters such as storage temperature, volume and thawing [27-29], probably explaining the frequent lack of correlation between labs using the same immunoassay kits.

Separately to CSF analysis, the research field has also developed a series of imaging approaches to assist clinical diagnosis such as Volumetric Magnetic Resonance Imaging (MRI) (to measure brain areas volume), FDG-PET and Amyloid PET imaging. Those are useful but currently provide only prognostic value to predict the likelihood to convert from MCI to AD [30, 31]. Amyloid PET tracers such as Pittsburgh Compound B and two new tracers, florbetapir-18 and flutemetamol-18, are approved as an *in vitro* diagnostic (IVD) but only to rule out possible AD pathology since a significant % of patients that test positive might never develop the disease [32]. Moreover, Positron Emission Tomography (PET) is very costly, and the scarcity of centers capable to handle this technology is still an issue in many countries. In UK, for example, only ~30 centers can perform this test, and the numbers are even lower in countries such as China [33]. These agents, although not reimbursed in US and other countries, are now proving useful to assist the development of novel drugs aiming to test the amyloid cascade hypothesis and are being used as enrollment criteria by several companies developing beta-secretase inhibitors as well as passive immunotherapies using anti-amyloid antibodies (Table 1). If these new therapies succeed, the availability of Amyloid-PET imaging as Companion Diagnostic (CDx) will still present the issues mentioned here as well as create additional economic burden on many healthcare systems. It is therefore accepted that having a first-line non-invasive diagnostic blood test comparable to Amyloid PET imaging would be precious in the clinical setting and could be used in tandem to diagnose patients correctly.

3. Recent progress in AD biomarker discoveries

3.1. Amyloid beta peptides and TAU in blood

Given the apparent association between Abeta accumulation and increase of P-TAU and Tau in brain and CSF of AD patients, several studies have looked at the change of Abeta 40/42 ratio in serum and plasma as non-invasive AD marker. At least 14 studies including our own that examined the change in such ratio in AD have been conducted [34] but have produced mixed results. It is not clear why such discrepancy is observed, but several factors not only related to patient's selection but also to assays themselves and how samples were stored and handled are possible explanations. It should be noted that even the Alzheimer's Disease Neuroimaging Initiative study (ADNI) data could not link Abeta40/42 plasma ratios to clinical state [35].What further complicate the use of plasma Abeta as an AD marker is the fact that it is produced not only centrally but also in the periphery and the nature itself of the peptide which tend to stick to walls and aggregate on itself affect the epitopes available during ELISA assays [34, 36].

Recently, researchers have also looked at Abeta 1-17 as a possible diagnostic marker of AD. One report showed that free-to-cell bound ratio of Abeta 1-17 could discriminate Control, MCI and AD patients with high sensitivity and specificity [37]. Additionally, plasma BACE1 enzyme, one key enzyme essential for the generation of Abeta peptides as well as soluble APP beta (sAPPbeta) have been found to be elevated in one study in AD patients plasma [38]. Despite the challenge of reliably measure Abeta 1-42 in plasma, a group demonstrated that APP669-711 appeared to be an indicator of pathological change of Abeta1-42. Ratio of APP669-711 to Abeta1-42 (APP669-711/Abeta1-42) measured by MALDI-TOF mass spectra showed a very good correlation with PIB+ signal in brain, suggesting that this plasma biomarker could be developed as a surrogate marker of cerebral amyloid deposition[39].

As for Tau and P-Tau detection in blood, demonstrating association with AD has been very challenging [40], especially for P-TAU due to the presence of circulating phosphatases in blood [24, 41] and the fact that TAU/P-TAU is elevated in multiple types of dementia including brain injuries [42]. A recent paper reporting the increase of an enzyme-generated fragment of TAU in serum that is inversely associated with cognitive function [43] seems promising. Another recently developed assay using antibodies reacting to all TAU isoforms could show with greater sensitivity than usual EIA methods the elevation of total Tau in serum of patients suffering from severe brain ischemia [44].Another group described the finding of oligomeric form of TAU in AD patients platelets [45] providing 76% sensitivity and 80% specificity. Time will tell if these TAU assays will be useful as a screening tool to support AD diagnosis.

3.2. Amyloid beta oligomers in blood

Amyloid beta (Aβ), especially Aβ42 oligomers play a significant role in early Alzheimer's disease (AD) pathogenesis [46, 47].In fact, AD-associated inflammation has been thought to be a secondary response to the pathological lesions triggered by Aβ oligomers in the early stage of pathogenesis. Although several studies, including our own (unpublished) have shown an elevation of such oligomers in CSF [48-52], few studies have looked at the correlation between blood oligomers concentration. In one study, levels of plasma Aβ monomers, Aβ oligomers, and soluble tumor necrosis factor α receptors (sTNFRs) were evaluated by ELISA in 120 controls, 32 amnestic mild cognitive impairment (aMCI) patients, and 90 mild AD patients [53]. The study found that levels of Aβ oligomers were significantly increased by ~two fold in mild AD patients compared to levels in aMCI and healthy controls. Interestingly, plasma levels of sTNFR in aMCI and mild AD patients was elevated significantly compared to controls, and both sTNFR1 and sTNFR2 levels were associated with levels of Aβ oligomers in both aMCI and mild AD individuals. Interestingly, changes in Aβ oligomer concentrations and sTNFR levels correctly differentiated mild ADfrom healthy control subjects.

In a separate study [50], another group have demonstrated that their ELISA system using BAN50 can detect signals in 60% of serum samples and 80% of CSF samples obtained from non-demented subjects.

individual peptide/ protein (plasma, serum)	comments	reference
Abeta 40/42 ratio	mixed results by various group	(34)
Abeta 1-17	free to bound cell ratio discriminate Control, MCI and AD	(37)
BACE1 enzyme, sAPPbeta	elevated in plasma	(38)
APP669-711/Abeta1-42	significant correlation with brain amyloid deposition (PIB+)	(39)
TAU fragment	level in serum inversely correlates with cognition deline	(42)
multiple TAU isoforms combination	elevated in patients suffering from brain ischemia	(43)
Oligomeric TAU	increase levels identified in platelets	(44)
Abeta oligomers (serum)	higher in MCI and AD subjects, not detected in all samples	(49, 52)
sTNFr	higher in MCI and AD subjects	(52)
proteins panels (plasma)		
30 serum proteins combination	set of several inflammatory and vascular related markers	(54, 55)
	combined with clinical data	
18 signalling plasma proteins combination	can differentiate AD and C, predict MCI conversion to AD	(56,57)
	(1 study could not reproduce this finding)	
Cortisol/VWF/oxidized LDL antibodies	can distinguish AD and C with 80% accuracy	(58)
Lipids (plasma)		
10 lipids combination	predicted phenoconversion from MCI to AD within 2-3 y	(61)
Ceramide/sphygomyelin	elevation correlates with MMSE score	(62)
Desmosterol/Cholesterol	decreased in MCI and AD, decrease % change in longitudinal cohorts	(66,73)
	correlates with rate of cognitive decline	
Genes, mRNAs, miRNAs		
96 genes signature (blood)	algorythm correctly predicts AD and discriminate Parkinson's Disease (CE mark test))	(75)
136 genes signature (blood)	algorythm identify AD patients over Controls (CE mark test)	(76)
48 genes signature (blood)	identify AD patients over Controls with even more accuracy when combined with MRI	(77)
TOMM40	expression in blood potentially useful to monitor AD progression/severity	(79)
98-5p,885-5p,483-3p,343-3p,191-5p,7d-5p	Asian population (Serum)	(131)
Let-7g-5p,142-3p,15b-5p,301s-3p,545-3p,191-5p,7d-5p	Caucasian population (Plasma)	(120)
7f,1285,107,103a-3p,26b-5p,26a-5p,532-5p,151a-3p,161,7d,112,5010-3p	Caucasian population (Whole blood cells)	(135)
miR-132,128,874,134,323-3p,382	Caucasian population (Plasma) (MCI correlation)	(109)
9,29a,29b,34a,125b,146a	Asian population (Plasma, CSF)	(158)
Others		
Two retinal amyloid depositions scans	detected after oral ingestion of curcumin tracer prior to eye scan using laser	AAIC 2014
	found good correlation with PIB amyloid positivity and/AV-45	O2-05-05
	ointment containing tracer applied to eye before laser scan	O3-12-01
Impairment of smell detection ability	association with brain region atrophy and prediction of conversion from MCI to AD	AAIC 2014

Table 2. Summary of non-invasive AD biomarker candidates

Although the levels of serum Abeta oligomers were reported to be unexpectedly high, the authors made the suggestion that the assay could be detecting non-pathological Abeta complexes associated with serum carrier proteins. Nonetheless, they did show a significant positive correlation with the levels obtained from matched CSF samples, suggesting that this assay system might be useful to support AD diagnosis.

4. Emerging blood-based AD biomarkers: Reproducibility of findings difficult

Novel non-invasive AD biomarkers found in blood are emerging as being a composition of different proteins, metabolites or gene transcripts in blood cells or single analytes. In total, there are as many as 21 literature studies in recent years looking at blood-based proteins association with AD. While the studies varied in size, they all looked at more than 100 proteins and the total number of patients examined ranged from 14 to 961, the 2 largest cohorts being ADNI (566) and AIBL (961). Kiddle et al. have recently published a report where they tried to replicate the findings of those 21 studies that linked a total of 163 proteins to AD using Somalogic's SOMAscan proteomics technology. 94 of those 163 candidate AD biomarkers were assessed in a relatively large cohorts of 677 subjects [54]. Only 9 candidate protein biomarkers were actually found to be related to at least 1 AD-related phenotypes: Pancreatic prohormone, Granulocyte colony-stimulating factor, Clusterin, Complement C3, Complement C6, Insulin-like growth factor-binding protein 2, Alpha-1-antitrypsin, inter-alpha-trypsin inhibitor heavy chain H4 and C-C motif chemokine 18. The outcome of this extensive replication study illustrates well the difficulty the field has been facing when trying to confirm previous findings in different patient cohorts.

5. Protein panel assays in development

Various protein panel assays have been developed by several groups with the use of algorithms to predict AD correctly. This approach is based on the assumption that combining markers together will increase the power of the test to identify patients correctly. One assay, in particular, is looking at 30 serum proteins and has 80% sensitivity and 91% specificity for diagnosing AD [55].The set of proteins is composed of several inflammatory and vascular related markers and the assay, combined with clinical data, showed a correlation with neuropsychological test performance [56].

Another group identified a panel of 18 signaling plasma proteins that can differentiate AD and control with ~90% sensitivity and identify MCI patients likely to convert to AD within 2 years with 81% sensitivity [57]. However, these results could not be reproduced independently [58].Combination of 3 blood markers (cortisol, von Willebrand factor and oxidized LDL antibodies) was able to diagnose AD with 80% accuracy [59].Quantitative mass-spectrometry-based selective reaction monitoring (SRM) is also supporting the development of AD diagnostic tests [60] by using isotopic tandem mass tag (TMT) technology to evaluate specific peptides derived from selected AD-related proteins. This approach, although very sound, is more difficult that one would think. In fact, when we tried in-house a similar technique called MRM (multiple reaction monitoring), we could not replicate several AD biomarker protein candidates discovered by other groups. Intriguingly, several peptides from the same protein showed changes in opposite directions (unpublished).

6. Plasma lipids as non-invasive AD biomarkers

The disturbance of several lipid pathways in the brain, in particular in cholesterol biosynthesis has been associated with several brain disorders including AD [61].So it comes as a little surprise that this category of molecule changes in blood to be another rich source of potential AD biomarkers. In a recent study, 525 community-dwelling healthy participants, aged 70 and older were enrolled as part of 5 year's observation study. Over the course of the study, 74 patients developed either MCI or mild AD. Using a lipidomic approach, the authors identified and validated a set of 10 lipids from peripheral blood that predicted phenoconversion to either MCI or AD within 2-3 year period with over 90% accuracy [62]. To our knowledge, this study is the first report of blood-based marker panel that can detect preclinical AD with such accuracy although validation using other cohorts will be required before considering clinical use. As the authors pointed out, alteration of lipids found in the cell membrane may be sensitive markers of neurodegeneration in pre-clinical AD. Another study using shotgun lipidomics, compared AD with controls individuals and found a change of ceramide/sphingomyelin ratio in AD [63] and its elevation to correlate with Mini-Mental-State-Examination scores (MMSE). This small study (26 AD and 26 controls) needs to be replicated though. Interestingly, a separate group found that an increase in this ratio was associated with slower disease progression [64]. Analysis of a longitudinal cohort of AD and control samples showed that AD patients had diminished baseline levels of either phospholipids, phosphatidylcholines, sphingomyelin and sterols as opposed to controls although they could not confirm the lipid profile to be good prognostic panel for estimating the progression to AD [65].

Our group initially discovered plasma desmosterol, the precursor of cholesterol, a metabolite that was recently identified as an LXR and RORgamma agonist[66, 67], as a candidate AD plasma marker [68]. Desmosterol is an essential sterol with hormone-like activity and account for as much as 30% of all brain sterols during most species brain development [69, 70].Multiple activities of desmosterol have also been reported, and it is understood that disturbances of the cholesterol metabolism may contribute to neurodegeneration [71, 72].

In our first study, decreased levels of desmosterol were observed (p value< 0.05, fold change= 0.36) in AD plasma samples versus controls plasma as well as in CSF [68]. Other groups also reported a decrease of desmosterol in brain as well as CSF [73] in an independent study but not in plasma. The discrepancy was understood in-house after we determined that this was due to an incomplete separation of cholesterol-desmosterol peaks during Gas Chromatography (AAIC 2012 abstract). Interestingly, we also observed a decrease of desmosterol also in

MCI and in particular, more pronounced in plasma of female AD patients plasma. This change of desmosterol in contrast was not affected by ApoE4 genotype. This finding was further validated and presented recently (AAIC 2013 abstract) using two large cohorts: a commercially available Caucasian sample set and a large Asian cohort. The Caucasian sample set consisted of a total of 109 patients (Control, MCI, and AD) and the large Asian cohort (n=401, 200 C and 201 AD) were both analyzed using LCMS. Our original data showing the association between decreased desmosterol/cholesterol ratio in AD and MCI was replicated in these cohorts. Data analysis showed that desmosterol level in plasma was found to be significantly different from AD and control groups with p-values 2.3E-14 and comparable AUC of ROC curve as initially found. High correlation between plasma desmosterol level and MMSE score was observed for these two large cohorts. As for novel AD candidate markers, we believe specificity should be investigated in other dementia types in order to understand the clinical usefulness of the marker and this work is currently on-going. In addition, the longitudinal analysis revealed that plasma Desmosterol/Cholesterol ratio (DES/CHO) in AD patients shows a significant decrease at follow-up intervals. The decline in plasma DES/CHO is larger in the AD group with rapid progression than in that with slow progression and the changes in plasma DES/CHO significantly correlated with changes in MMSE score.

Altogether, this data means that plasma DES/CHO decrease in AD patients may serve as a longitudinal surrogate marker associated with cognitive decline. This data, as well as an additional longitudinal cohort data analysis, is now in press at the time of this writing[74].

Very interestingly, a minor allele of an intronic SNP within DHCR24 gene (the gene coding for the protein responsible to convert desmosterol into cholesterol) was identified in a recent ADNI study and was associated with a lower average PiB PET uptake, a first generation imaging amyloid PET agent that is used to understand amyloid deposit load in AD brain [75].It is tempting to speculate that lower desmosterol levels in the brain (reflected as well in plasma and CSF) could be directly linked to higher amyloid deposition.

In order to further understand the utility of desmosterol as an AD biomarker, we collected patients plasma samples obtained through one of our ongoing AD clinical phase 2 trial, that were either positive or negative on Amyloid Pet scans (Flurbetamol) and data analysis is now ongoing. Possible outcome of this study could help patient stratification in further trials and lead to the development of a first line test prior to conducting more expensive PET imaging scans for patients enrolment in future trials or to the development of a stand-alone *in vitro* diagnostics.

7. Genes, mRNA, and miRNAs

Because gene transcription and translation ultimately determine the production of proteins that regulate cells and tissue functions, several groups have been looking at molecular changes in AD vs Controls in blood components and circulating peripheral cells to identify biomarkers. Among these, one group looked at the expression of 96 different genes in blood. A whole genome analysis was conducted using oligonucleotide microarray and blood from a large clinical cohort consisting of AD patients and control healthy subjects. a. Gene analysis comparing the gene expression of 94 AD patients and 94 cognitive healthy controls was conducted, and a disease classifier algorithm developed [76].

Validation was conducted on an independent cohort consisting of 63 subjects that included 50% AD patients,40% aged-matched controls and 10% young healthy controls. The results showed the test to have an accuracy of 87% to predict AD pathology. Additionally, the algorithm also discriminated AD from Parkinson's disease in 24/27 patients (accuracy 89%).

Another group developed an alternate gene AD signature consisting of 136 different genes using 177 blood samples (90 AD patients and 87 controls) [77]. Signature validation was then later performed on a blinded independent cohort of 209 individuals (111 AD and 98 controls). Many of the genes included in the signature are found to be elevated during inflammation processes and apoptosis and have been associated with the amyloid cascade and tau pathology. In a follow-up validation study consisting of 164 patients.. This test performed relatively well and was able to identify AD patients (81.3% sensitivity) correctly and to exclude AD pathology (67.1% specificity). Both of these tests have won approval in Europe (CE Mark) as AD biomarker and are available to physicians but they still haven't been validated in large clinical cohorts such as the Alzheimer's Disease Neuroimaging Initiative (ADNI ½).

At least two other studies showed this transcriptome approach potential. In one study [78], a gene expression signature was discovered in a 156 patients cohorts consisting of AD and controls. The validation study confirmed the performance of the gene signature in a separate cohort composed of 26 AD, 26 healthy age-matched control and 118 mild MCI individuals classified as probable early AD subjects. The 48 genes signature accurately identified 70% of AD patients and when combined with MRI defined criteria, the accuracy went up to 85%.,. However, the authors indicated that these results have to be validated in other diseases or dementias.

The same group also looked at changes in gene expression in leukocytes and found alterations in blood seen mild cognitive impairment (MCI) and AD subjects indicating a peripheral response to pathology may occur very early [79].Noticeably, evidences for mitochondrial dysfunction indicated by a reduce expression of several respiratory complex I-V genes were observed, confirming changes previously seen in AD brain.

One novel single gene marker identified that is associated with AD is TOMM40 (translocase of outer mitochondrial membrane 40 homolog). The protein encoded by TOMM40 seems to transport proteins functionally to mitochondria. Risk Mutation in this gene has been found in several GWAS studies, and one group showed that its expression in blood may serve as an AD marker of disease severity and progression [80].

8. miRNAs

Beside the existing proteomic, metabolomics and nucleic acid based markers, small RNAs (including miRNAs) are an upcoming class of circulating biomarkers that have resulted in many new findings. miRNAs belong to the class of non-coding regulatory RNA molecules of ~22nt length that regulate gene expression post-transcriptionally by binding (in most cases) to the 3' un-translated region (UTRs) of their targets [81-83]. It is estimated that ~5% genes in the human genome encode for miRNAs and a single miRNA can regulate multiple targets (sometimes in excess of 200) based primarily on the complementarity of the seed region (nt 2-8 of the miRNA) to target mRNA molecules [84]. MicroRNAs play regulatory roles in vital biological processes, including cell proliferation and growth, tissue differentiation, development, and cell death[85]. Interestingly, it has recently been demonstrated, that not only are miRNAs active in their cell of origin, but they can be exported/secreted out, and cause down-regulation of target mRNAs in an alternate target cell [86]. It is this unique property of miRNAs of being present in intact and functional condition in circulating biofluids including CSF, plasma, serum, urine, tears and saliva, which makes them promising biomarker candidates. They are found enclosed in membrane-bound structures (exosomes, microvesicles etc.) [87, 88], and in some cases in "free" form, protected by RNA binding proteins like NPM1, HDL [86, 89] or Argonaute2 [90, 91]. Circulating miRNA signatures have been shown to identify different tumor types [92, 93] indicate staging and progression of the disease [94] and serve as prognostic markers [95, 96]. Recently, five miRNA based diagnostic tests have been made available for clinicians to prescribe (through Rosetta Genomics and Asuragen Inc). Although the first generation of tests requires tumor biopsies, there is now significant work in progress to eliminate the need for getting biopsies, and to be able to get answers from blood, urine or other readily available circulating fluids.

Although the potential of miRNAs as diagnostic markers has been consistently demonstrated in Oncology; recent publications in other areas like neurodegenerative disorders point to their expanding role [99]. In AD, for example, miRNA profiling experiments (in brain tissue) have resulted in the identification of many disease-specific miRNAs that have been confirmed independently in two or more studies [97]. For example, hsa-miR-106, hsa-miR-153 and hsa-miR-101 have been shown to modulate APP [98-101], while BACE1 has been shown to be targeted by hsa-miRNA-29 and hsa-miR-107, linking miRNAs to regulation of amyloid production in AD brains [102]. Based on similar studies, researchers have focused on these disease-specific miRNAs to determine if differential levels are found in more-easily accessible biofluids like blood or CSF. Hsa-miR-29a/b including others was a disease-specific miRNA whose down-regulated levels in the serum of AD patients mimicked the expected down-regulation in the brain tissue [103]. This is a more disease-focused approach, where only those miRNAs that have a known link to the illness is profiled for. However, the nature of circulating fluids, which allows all organs, tissues to be potential sources of biomarkers makes a simple correlation with only diseased focus biomarkers (miRNAs, in this case) hard. There is also now a confirmed presence of a selective gating mechanism that determines a particular profile of miRNAs to be exported out (in exosomes or protein bound). This was recently demonstrated in studies that showed that secreted miRNA profiles (from culture) were not in correlation with intra-cellular profiles. This could explain why higher level of a miRNA in an affected organ is not automatically associated with an increase in its plasma level [104, 105]. Another approach, still under the umbrella of disease-relevant miRNAs looks not at the disease etiology, but broadens the net and looks for all miRNAs known to be expressed in the tissue/

organ of interest. Hence for AD for examples, miRNAs known to be enriched in neurons and synapse destruction were focused on [109-111]. As a result, miR-132 and the miR-134 family of miRNAs were discovered which showed potential for differentiation between MCI and AD, and, in fact, could also predict 1-5 years in advance of a clinical diagnosis. Potential biomarkers like these could be instrumental in identifying the population which would respond best to therapy in the future, or at least identify the correct pool of patients who are MCI for example, but would advance to AD in the absence of any treatment. On the Neurodegeneration side, some focused miRNA analysis has uncovered candidates like miR-146a and miR-155 that were found in higher levels in brain tissue extra-cellular fluid (ECF) in AD patients [112]. Along with the recent report on let-7b that is being investigated as a TLR-7 ligand [113], these recent findings point towards the potential role of inflammation, which ultimately could lead to neurodegenerative disorders.

Without limiting the miRNA profiles to either disease etiology or organ/tissue of focus, unbiased-global profiling is another approach to biomarker research. This is now especially more feasible, considering the significant technological advancements that have allowed researchers to look at thousands of biomarkers using as little as 100 ul of blood, for example. Another reason, why an unbiased approach might be appealing to certain researchers is the potential of finding novel pathways that have so far not been implicated in the disease of interest, and this is especially true for complex, heterogeneous disorders like AD, where there is still a lot of work on going in trying to understand all the biology of the disease. Of course, on the flip-side, it is often difficult to explain the biological significance and connection of the novel biomarker for the illness. The problem is more severe for miRNAs, because it is not a simple miRNA-mRNA relationship, but rather a single miRNA, and hundreds of potential mRNA targets [114-116], which makes it even harder to predict connections to disease. To put this conundrum of multiple miRNA targets into a biological context, this publication proposed [117] that usually biologically meaningful targets of miRNAs were found to be enriched in specific pathways, or a network. The first un-biased miRNA study in blood (PBMCs) was done in 2007 [106] followed by a much-cited study by Cogswell et al.[107] that identified miRNAs differentially expressed in brain and CFS of AD/matched controls. In addition to some related pathways being implicated in neuronal differentiation and actin remodeling (through targets of miR-9 and 132), novel target pathways like brain insulin signaling and oxidative stress were identified. However, the surprise finding was the lack of correlation between CSF and brain profiles, which again hinted at a particular secretion mechanism that regulated the transfer of miRNAs from the cell. In addition, differentially expressed CSF miRNAa like miR-146b (thought to be involved in immune function) were found to be decreased in AD patients, suggesting an activated immune status, potentially offering insights into the role of inflammation in the disease.

Consistent with the global profiling approach, our group had published a novel AD signature that had >95% accuracy in determining AD status from matched controls [108]. It consisted of reduced levels of 7 miRNAs (hsa-let-7d-5p, hsa-let-7g-5p, hsa-miR-15b-5p, hsa-miR-142-3p, hsa-miR-191-5p, hsa-miR-301a-3p and hsa-miR-545-3p) which was further confirmed in an independent sample-set of 20 AD and 17 NC samples, To put a biological context to the hundreds of potential miRNA target molecules, we enriched for mRNA molecules that were targeted by multiple miRNAs (at least 2) Some neurological canonical pathways identified included axonal guidance signaling, ephrin receptor signaling [109], actin cytoskeleton signaling[110], clathrin-mediated endocytosis signaling [111] and RhoA signaling [112]. These pathways, although diverse, show potential biological relationships with disease etiology [125]. Using an unbiased analysis approach, we removed the filter of neurological pathways in IPA, and got a list of pathways enriched for signature miRNA targets., A type II Diabetes Mellitus signaling canonical pathway was identified. This was interesting because there was also evidence from multiple GWAS studies indicating that SNPs in ApoE [113] Clu [114] and ABCA7 genes [115] were linked to AD biology. This was in addition to another report that linked lipid metabolism to both amyloid and tau pathology [61]. However, due to unclear outcomes after statin treatment in AD clinical trials, the role of lipid metabolism in AD pathogenesis remains to be elucidated [116]. In another global-approach driven study in serum, miRNAs were profiled from 50 AD and 50 matched control samples using next-generation sequencing [117] This was followed by a validation study using qRT-PCR in an independent cohort of 158 AD and 155 control populations. Amongst other signature miRNAs identified, miR-191-5p and let-7d-5p were identified to be down-regulated in AD patients. This was encouraging because it validated part of our miRNA signature in blood (serum) using a different profiling technology (NGS) as opposed to a hybridization-based technology (nCounter: Nanostring) used by our group. This suggested that the signature had biological relevance and was not likely a profiling or normalization artifact, which often results in little validation rates of miRNA signatures.

Having previously established that the signature miRNAs could reliably differentiate AD from a matched control population NC, we investigated if lower levels of these miRNAs could be observed at earlier stages of dementia. To address this, a new set of samples containing 27 AD, 30 MCI, and 59 NC samples was obtained. All 7signature miRNAs were confirmed to be differentially expressed between the new cohort of 27 AD and 59 NC samples (internal data, not published). In addition, these miRNAs could reliably differentiate between MCI and NC samples. Meanwhile, no significant difference was observed between MCI and AD samples. To eliminate a potential normalization bias because of our choice of normalization strategy (geometric mean of ath-159a and hsa-miR-106), the data was normalized in two additional ways. The geometric mean of hsa-miR-16-5p and ath-miR-159a was used for normalization, given previous use of hsa-miR-16 as the miRNA of choice for normalization for plasma-based miRNA profiles [118, 119]. In addition, spike-in ath-159a was used in isolation to account for the possibility that normalization with endogenous control miRNAs might prevent detection of valid and meaningful biological variation. We observed no significant change in fold-changes or p –values for AD/NC and MCI/NC confirming that the signature was robust and not sensitive to different normalization strategies. Inter-site reproducibility was also investigated and an aliquot of total RNA was tested at another site by a different operator following the described protocol. Excellent correlations were observed for all 7-miRNA signatures, demonstrating the robustness of the entire assay workflow.

It was encouraging, that the same signature set of miRNAs that could differentiate AD from NC individuals was also downregulated in MCI patients. This suggested that these signature miRNAs were potentially related to early events in the disease and could be valuable for the early identification of AD/MCI patients for potential stratification in clinical studies. However, care should be exercised in how one interpret these findings. Patients that have been diagnosed as MCI are a heterogeneous population, which can have very diverse outcomes as a result of their MCI diagnosis. Some patients continue in the MCI phase or advance to more severe MCI states while, for others, conditions might deteriorate towards dementia. While some MCI patients go on to develop dementia linked to Frontal Temporal Lobe Dementia (FTLD) or Dementia with Lewy Bodies (DLB), a majority of patients develop dementia driven by pathophysiological processes attributed to Alzheimer's with a conversion rate of ~15-20% per year [120] So it is important to follow up with more studies to understand the course of progression for the MCI population tested, and evaluate if we can predict conversion of MCI to AD (for example) using this signature set of miRNAs. In addition to the specificity of any diagnostic signature for Alzheimer's disease, determining how early in disease etiology the biomarker in question changes is also critical. Archived samples are going back years before the actual diagnosis of MCI or AD would need to be accessed and processed to understand the timing of the biomarker aberration. For a biomarker signature to be valuable for a longitudinal evaluation, it is helpful to comprehend the variation and stability of the proposed biomarker across time. We observed an average coefficient of variation between 15 and 25% for 6 out of 7 miRNAs for eight healthy individuals across samples taken from multiple 6-month visits spread over 3-4 years (unpublished). This set of data indicates that the signature miRNAs are indeed stable across time in individuals, and are therefore promising candidates to evaluate in longitudinal samples from individual patients to understand at what point, these biomarkers start to change (in Alzheimer's progression, for example).

In another global, unbiased study, researchers looked at whole blood cells from Alzheimer's and age-matched control samples to discover diagnostic miRNA signatures. They utilized a next-generation-sequencing platform for profiling the miRNAs in a discovery cohort of 48 AD and 22 unaffected control samples, while the validation was done using qRT-PCR in a larger cohort of over 200 patients comprising not only of AD patients but also patients suffering from other CNS illnesses. They achieved a 12-miRNA signature, which had an accuracy of 93% to differentiate AD from matched control samples [121] The accuracy was significantly lower (74-78%) to distinguish AD from other CNS disorders. In another study, researchers looked at profiling serum samples from 22 AD and control samples, which comprised of 18 non-inflammatory neurological disease controls (NINDCs) and eight inflammatory neurological disease controls (INDCs). Although they used an unbiased approach and did not restrict the number of miRNAs to disease-associated candidates, they only profiled the most abundantly expressed miRNAs (a panel of 192 miRNAs), and then followed up with qRT-PCR validation. MicroRNA-125b and miR-26b were found to be down-regulated in AD, and confirmed in CSF from the same patient population [122] Accuracy was determined to be 82% for differentiating between AD and NINDC cohorts. Although they had an FTD cohort (Frontotemporal Lobe Dementia), the number of patients was too small [10] to make significant conclusions about the specificity of the signature.

While there is a lot of activities, excitement, and hope for a non-invasive, specific, cost effective and quantitative biomarker for early detection of Alzheimer's, there has also been a concerning lack of concordance reported amongst individual studies trying to reproduce previous signatures for Alzheimer's (Fig. 2). This is true for miRNA signatures for other diseases as well. A number of unique, independent signatures, especially for Oncology have been reported previously [123] but most of them remained un-validated or never progressed to the clinic stage. There are several reasons for this. Throughout the process of miRNA profiling and subsequent validation, there are steps in which individual biases get introduced, which are unique to each profiling method. The choice of starting material, be it plasma, serum, whole blood cells, PBMC's, or even exosomes from the blood impact signature profiles. The extraction method is another source of variation, as evidenced by the recent retraction[124], where it was reported that Trizol based preparations were susceptible to non-uniform extraction biases depending on initial concentration of certain miRNAs (with particular GC content profiles) in the sample. Gender, ethnicity, age [125] are some other factors that are known to affect miRNA profiles. Hence if one study utilized a defined cohort of patients that were Caucasian in ethnicity, while another group tried to replicate the signature in a cohort that was mixed with Hispanic or African American patient samples, concordance between the two studies could be compromised There has also been considerable concern about presence of blood-cell derived miRNAs that are found in the plasma fraction, occurring because of hemolysis of blood cells during plasma preparation [126, 127]. Hence, subtle differences in plasma preparation methods could impact plasma signatures significantly. Platelet contamination during plasma preparation is another source of potential discordance [128]. Even in our study, we have observed center to center variation and now more work needs to be done in identifying the source of variation, be it plasma handling leading to platelet contamination from some centers, or the effect of platelet activation leading to microparticle shedding, which also could impact the miRNA signature performance.

Post sample preparation, the choice of profiling platform utilized for discovery and validation has a significant effect on miRNA levels. A study compared biases in miRNA profiling across hybridization-based array platforms and a Next Generation Sequencing (NGS) platform [129] AU-rich miRNAs were detected with higher sensitivity using NGS based platforms; while GC-rich miRNAs were preferably detected using Hybridization based array platforms. Within a NGS platform itself, biases for certain miRNAs exist, that are driven by sequence (3`nt) and secondary structure at the ligation site [130] of individual miRNAs and adapters, affecting ligase enzyme efficiency during the library construction step. What further compounds the issue is that typically after discovery using a high-throughput platform, miRNA signatures are usually validated using qPCR based methods, which adds their bias to the analysis. Stem loop RT-PCR primers, that are often the "gold standard" for miRNA detection only bind to the 3' 8-10 nt of the miRNA in question, and hence are susceptible to stable secondary structures at the 3' end of miRNAs that inhibit efficient primer initiation in the typical temperature range of reverse transcription (37° to 42°C). Alternatively, with the LNA (modified primers using Locked Nucleic Acid modifications to increase the Tm of smaller sized primers to accommo-date size limitations of miRNAs method, polyadenylation is used to elongate the short miRNA sequence, followed by RT-qPCR detection. Due to substrate preferences and secondary structures at the 3′ end of the miRNA, certain miRNAs are better substrates than others for this first step, causing a bias. A recent analysis published in Nature captured the variability in miRNA profiling platforms [131]. They evaluated up to 12 profiling platforms using standardized sample sets. The platforms were PCR, hybridization or sequencing based. As expected, the PCR-based platforms resulted in higher sensitivity, although sometimes at a cost of accuracy and specificity. Metrics tested included reproducibility, dynamic range performance, accuracy, accuracy at lower RNA input, sensitivity, sensitivity at a lower RNA input specificity and cross assay reactivity. The lower volume metrics were designed to address applications like detection of circulating miRNAs from body fluids, where the concentrations of miRNAs are typically very small. Although differences were expected between platforms, what was surprising was the extent of discordance observed between platforms. The average validation rate between any two platforms was as low as 54%. This labors the point, that it is paramount to profile and validate using two different platforms to confirm potential signature miRNAs in order to eliminate platform artifacts. Moreover, lastly, the multiple normalization strategies that are used for circulating miRNA analysis further reduce concordance between independent studies. Because of a lack of a well-established and accepted normalization miRNA candidate (a GAPDH equivalent for miRNAs), there have been a variety of strategies utilized and have been previously reviewed [132, 133]. Each approach makes certain assumptions, and it is important to consider those when comparing different miRNA profiling studies. Given these above mentioned sources of variation, it is not surprising that multiple studies which started in 2007, where miRNAs were profiled using microarray technologies (that modified mRNA based strategies to work with the much shorter miRNAs) to today, where you have the next generation of technologies that have been built keeping miRNAs in mind, the miRNA profiles are significantly different. Furthermore, there have been constant additions/subtractions and even sequence edits to the miRBASE registry over the years, which have an impact on profiling platforms, since they have to modify probes in order to accommodate these changes. With the recent discovery and advancement in technologies to look at exosomes, another dimension of complexity has been added, where one can distinguish exosome encapsulated fractions and truly cell-free fractions, further reducing concordance between studies. Hence it is important to maintain very standard protocols, and then follow through with them till the end of the study, including multiple validations with many independent cohorts of samples taken from different centers, ethnicities and ages.

The last 3-4 years have seen the beginning of the utilization of circulating miRNAs in the neurodegenerative disorders domain, and it is still a maturing field. The potential of miRNAs to provide a cost effective, non-invasive, accurate and sensitive diagnostic assay resulting in a positive impact on patient health is undeniable, but care needs to be exercised in interpretation of these signatures in the absence of thorough validation. Furthermore, significant work detailing how these novel biomarkers tie into disease etiology is a must to increase confidence and understand the reason behind biomarker modulation due to illness or subsequent treatment.

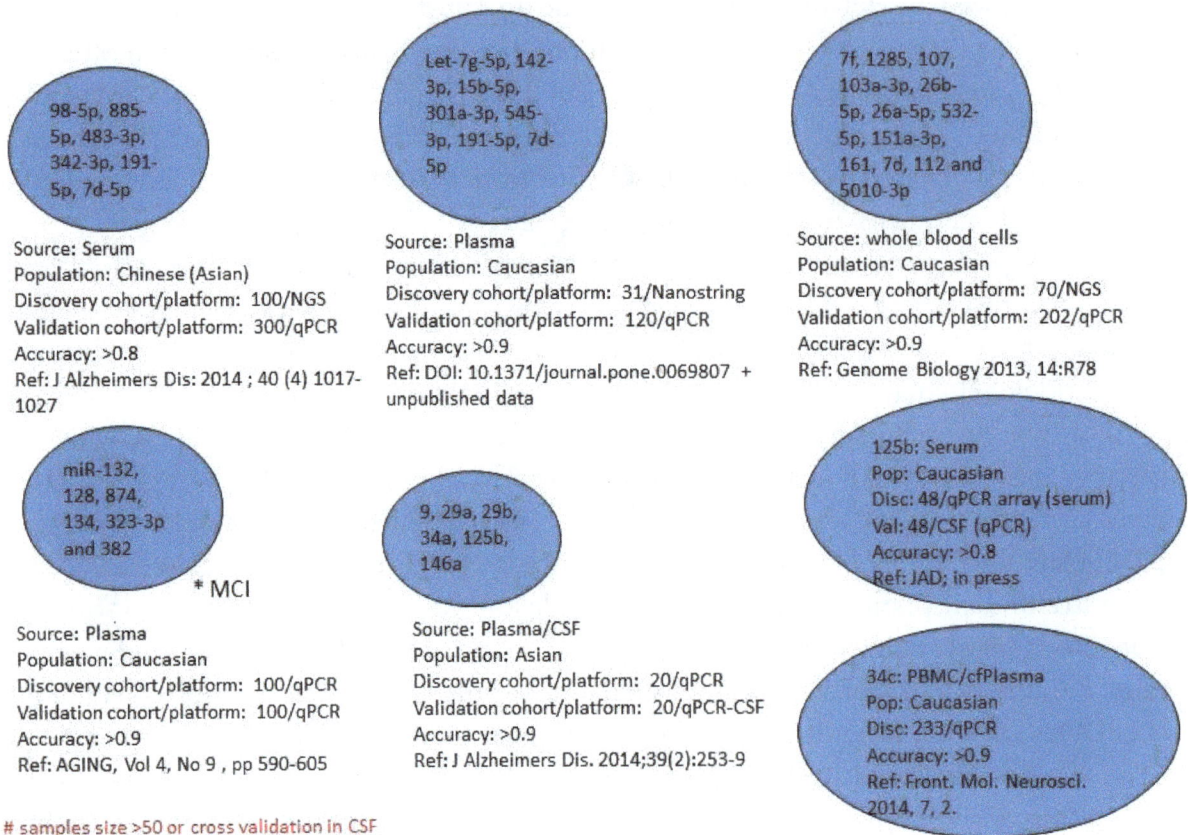

Figure 2. Snapshot of current circulating miRNA signatures# for Alzheimer's Disease

9. New non-invasive biomarkers on the horizon

Despite the promising collection of novel blood-based biomarkers as we just described, there is still a possibility to unravel additional novel non-invasive biomarkers for AD and MCI in other accessible body matrices. The human retina shares many features with the brain, including embryological origin, anatomical (ex. Microvasculature bed) and important physiological characteristics such as blood-tissue barrier [134] So researchers have looked at the possibility that the retina may offer an easily accessible and non-invasive way of examining human brain pathology. As it turned out, it is becoming evident that amyloid is also accumulating in the eyes and that this landmark event could be detected by relatively straightforward eye examinations according to data derived from multiple research trials data presented during the summer of 2014 at the Alzheimer's Association International Conference held in Copenhagen.. Data from independent studies showed that the level of beta-amyloid detected in the eye was significantly correlated with the level of beta-amyloid deposition in the brain and allowed researchers to accurately identify patients with Alzheimer's in the studies.

In the first study looking at healthy patients from the Australian Imaging, Biomarker and Lifestyle Flagship Stud Preliminary data from the first 40 participants showed that amyloid levels detected in the retina using an orally administered curcumin supplement were significantly correlated with brain amyloid levels, as shown by PiB PET imaging. In addition, Retinal Amyloid Imaging (RAI) differentiated participants with AD from those without AD with 100% sensitivity and 80.6% specificity. Furthermore, longitudinal data showed a 3.5% elevation on average in retinal amyloid signal during a 3.5-month period, suggesting that the technique may be used as a means of monitoring response to therapy.

The second separate phase 2 studies included 20 individuals with probable mild to moderate AD and 20 healthy, age-matched control participants. In this study, participants had a small proprietary molecule applied to the eye in the form of a sterile ophthalmic ointment. The compound was left to diffuse into the eye overnight and the next day the eye was scanned with the laser and results computed. As in the first study, all 40 participants also underwent PET amyloid brain imaging but this time with Amyvid PET agent. The test was capable to distinguish individuals with Alzheimer's from healthy control participants with 85% sensitivity and 95% specificity significantly and as in the first study, amyloid levels in the lens significantly correlated with PET imaging results.

Given the rapidity and simplicity of the diagnostic test (5 minutes) it is easy to understand how revolutionary this would be for the medical field as it could be used by general practitioners and specialists at point-of-care in hospitals and offices. Time will tell if it could also be used to monitor disease progression and monitor efficacy of new anti-Alzheimer's drug in development (Alzheimer's Association International Conference (AAIC) 2014. Abstracts O2-05-05 and O3-13-01).

10. Impairment of odor detection as early AD diagnostic

It is becoming evident that as AD sets in, impairment of the olfaction system in its ability to correctly distinguish odors appears to be an early phenomenon that could predict cognitive impairment at an early stage (AAIC 2014, in Copenhagen). In two studies, the decreased ability to identify various defined odors was significantly associated with loss of neuronal cells function and progression to Alzheimer's disease as measured by a variety of cognitive tests.

Imaging data from one study revealed that a smaller hippocampus and a thinner entorhinal cortex accompanied by higher levels of brain amyloid were linked to worsening of smell identification abilities and memory after adjusting for parameters that includes age, gender, and an estimate of cognitive reserve(AAIC 2014).

A separate study conducted at Columbia University Medical Center looked at odor Identification deficits association with Transition from Mild Cognitive Impairment to Alzheimer's. Researchers investigated a multi-ethnic sample of 1037 non-demented elderly people in New York City, (average age of 80.7) and assessed their olfaction abilities in a variety of ways at three time periods. 109 people developed dementia (101=Alzheimer's and eight non-AD dementia) a significant incapacity to correctly identify odors was found to be associated with the early development of dementia in those patients.

Although further large-scale studies will be required to confirm these results it is encouraging for the medical practice field that such relatively inexpensive test may be used one day to detect early stage of AD and those at risk of cognitive decline.

11. Urine

There are very few reports describing the discovery of any AD-related urine biomarker, and the few that are reported and published have met the AD research field with controversy. One of them is called NTP (Neural Thread Protein), a membrane-associated phosphoprotein that made the headlines in 2007 when a company called Nymox Corporation got an EIA kit CE approved in Europe for the diagnosis of AD using urine samples. Although Nymox claimed the utility of the test, one blinded study conducted in the Czech Republic by a reference lab using the Nymox test found that when compared to the diagnosis established by NINCDS-ADRDA for AD, the test appeared to have low sensitivity and specificity. Very recently, two studies evaluating the levels of NTP in urine were published [135, 136]. In the first study, levels of NTP in AD, PD, and Healthy participants were evaluated (AD (49, PD (20), HC (22) using Nymox AlzhemAlert test. AD patients had significantly higher levels of NTP than HC and that those of PD. Although the authors concluded that urine NTP could be used as a promising biomarker of AD, it should be noted that there was an age difference among participants that could potentially affect this interpretation. Average age for each group was as follows: AD (72.2+/-7.5), PD (66.4 +/- 8.8), Control (64.1+/-6.8).

In a second separate recent study [137], NTP levels were compared in relation to age in HC volunteers divided into 5 groups (20-29, 30-39,40-49,50-59 and >=60) using a different test called 7c Gold..It is not clear as to why the levels detected in this study are in ng/ml range as opposed to the ug/ml range for the Nymox Kit since both studies were conducted on Asian patients. The authors concluded though that urine levels of NTP increase with age significantly which might explain the controversy around NTP as an AD biomarker.

12. Conclusion

12.1. Hurdles to blood-based AD biomarker development

Replicating candidate blood biomarker findings has been the biggest challenge of the research field [138]. Several pre-analytical components factors are likely to make discoveries very challenging: choice of anticoagulant (EDTA, Heparin), addition of protease inhibitors, needle size, order of blood draw, processing time, storage condition, freeze/thaw cycles and centrifugation procedures are just a few parameters that can affect drastically the detection of several analytes [128, 138]. Longitudinal analysis from the same patient is essential to find early markers, but the success of this approach highly depends on analyte stability during >10 years storage. Blood is also a constantly changing matrix where components levels are affected by multiple factors such as diet, lifestyle, circadian changes and other co-morbidities, especially in an elderly population such as Alzheimer's Disease patients which quite frequently suffers from other diseases where inflammation is implicated such as diabetes, rheumatoid arthritis and cardiovascular diseases [139].Further complicating discoveries is the fact that several patients have mixed dementias such as Vascular Dementia, Fronto Temporal Lobe Dementia (FTLD) and Dementia with Lewy-body (DLB) making it difficult to identify a particular marker. Importantly, the integrity of the blood-brain barrier and its impact on AD-related biomarkers might differ from patient to patient based on genetics and other factors [140].Another less discussed parameter that we found that is crucial for the discovery of true AD blood biomarkers is the definition of healthy controls. We realized talking to clinical physicians in Japan, US, and EU that in many instances, healthy elderly control samples are obtained from caregivers or spouses living with the patients. This is a particular concern since epidemiological studies have demonstrated that living with an AD patient increases the risk to develop the disease by six-fold [141]. The reason is not exactly known but contributing factors such as exposure to pollutants (air, water, contaminants in food, etc) and pathogens [142, 143] by the patient and the spouse for several years living in the same environment may play a role. We also heard through interviews with clinicians that several healthy control samples are obtained from patients who went to a clinic after complaining of some abnormalities that were later ruled out as not being related to dementia. The inclusion of such patient samples in the control group category may also contribute to the difficulty of identifying a true AD biomarker.

While co-morbidities cannot be avoided when comparing AD and control groups, it is important to the research field to agree on standard practices to ensure reproducibility of data and that careful selection of healthy controls be conducted before doing any comparisons. At least, initiatives like the Blood-Based Biomarker Interest Group and the release of FDA guidelines for the analytical validation of assays that meet GCP/GLP will hopefully lead to the adoption of robust standards for the research field that applies to the analysis of proteins, metabolites, lipids and miRNAs in serum and plasma to control for precision, analytical accuracy and dilution linearity.

One more important point for the successful development and adoption of blood-based AD biomarkers is to understand the relationship with the disease as AD is essentially a brain disorder with little manifestation of illness in the peripheral system. Such understanding of the biomarker, its function, and its contribution to the illness state is essential to promote the confirmation by peers. Moreover, such clarification could lead to the discovery of even better biomarkers that could be used to detect the disease at an even earlier state or lead to the identification of novel drug targets. Such functional identification as much as the validation is critical to promote the verification of novel candidate biomarker in exploratory studies that are part of sponsored clinical trials.

In conclusion, blood tests or other non-invasive tests as biomarkers for AD are appealing as they could be applied to many uses such as patient screening, disease prognosis, diagnosis and aid to support clinical trial development. The development of such markers will be greatly facilitated once we fully understand what is causing sporadic AD in the first place and after more comprehensive studies will be able to look at correlation between endophenotypic changes in the brain using imaging technologies and the candidate biomarkers.

Author details

Francois Bernier[1], Pavan Kumar[2], Yoshiaki Sato[1] and Yoshiya Oda[1,2*]

*Address all correspondence to: yoshiya_oda@eisai.com

1 Eisai Co., Ltd., Tokodai, Tsukuba, Ibaraki, Japan

2 Eisai IncAndover, MA, USA

References

[1] Cummings JL, Morstorf T, Zhong K. Alzheimer's disease drug-development pipeline: few candidates, frequent failures. Alzheimers Res Ther. 2014;6(4):37.

[2] Hardy JA, Higgins GA. Alzheimer's disease: the amyloid cascade hypothesis. Science. 1992 Apr 10;256(5054):184-5.

[3] Rushworth JV, Griffiths HH, Watt NT, Hooper NM. Prion protein-mediated toxicity of amyloid-beta oligomers requires lipid rafts and the transmembrane LRP1. J Biol Chem. 2013 Mar 29;288(13):8935-51.

[4] Abisambra JF, Scheff S. Brain injury in the context of tauopathies. J Alzheimers Dis. 2014;40(3):495-518.

[5] Krstic D, Knuesel I. Deciphering the mechanism underlying late-onset Alzheimer disease. Nat Rev Neurol. 2013 Jan;9(1):25-34.

[6] Jack CR, Jr., Knopman DS, Jagust WJ, Petersen RC, Weiner MW, Aisen PS, et al. Tracking pathophysiological processes in Alzheimer's disease: an updated hypothetical model of dynamic biomarkers. Lancet Neurol. 2013 Feb;12(2):207-16.

[7] Henley DB, Sundell KL, Sethuraman G, Dowsett SA, May PC. Safety profile of semagacestat, a gamma-secretase inhibitor: IDENTITY trial findings. Curr Med Res Opin. 2014 Jul 14:1-12.

[8] Lannfelt L, Relkin NR, Siemers ER. Amyloid-ss-directed immunotherapy for Alzheimer's disease. J Intern Med. 2014 Mar;275(3):284-95.

[9] Counts SE, Lahiri DK. Editorial: Overview of Immunotherapy in Alzheimer's Disease (AD) and Mechanisms of IVIG Neuroprotection in Preclinical Models of AD. Curr Alzheimer Res. 2014;11(7):623-5.

[10] Wisniewski T, Goni F. Immunotherapy for Alzheimer's disease. Biochem Pharmacol. 2014 Apr 15;88(4):499-507.

[11] Salloway S, Sperling R, Fox NC, Blennow K, Klunk W, Raskind M, et al. Two phase 3 trials of bapineuzumab in mild-to-moderate Alzheimer's disease. N Engl J Med. 2014 Jan 23;370(4):322-33.

[12] Doody RS, Thomas RG, Farlow M, Iwatsubo T, Vellas B, Joffe S, et al. Phase 3 trials of solanezumab for mild-to-moderate Alzheimer's disease. N Engl J Med. 2014 Jan 23;370(4):311-21.

[13] Grimmer T, Wutz C, Drzezga A, Forster S, Forstl H, Ortner M, et al. The usefulness of amyloid imaging in predicting the clinical outcome after two years in subjects with mild cognitive impairment. Curr Alzheimer Res. 2013 Jan;10(1):82-5.

[14] Okello A, Koivunen J, Edison P, Archer HA, Turkheimer FE, Nagren K, et al. Conversion of amyloid positive and negative MCI to AD over 3 years: an 11C-PIB PET study. Neurology. 2009 Sep 8;73(10):754-60.

[15] Weiner MW. Commentary on "Biomarkers in Alzheimer's disease drug development." The view from Alzheimer's Disease Neuroimaging Initiative. Alzheimers Dement. 2011 May;7(3):e45-7.

[16] Mitka M. PET imaging for Alzheimer disease: are its benefits worth the cost? JAMA. 2013 Mar 20;309(11):1099-100.

[17] Lorenzi M, Donohue M, Paternico D, Scarpazza C, Ostrowitzki S, Blin O, et al. Enrichment through biomarkers in clinical trials of Alzheimer's drugs in patients with mild cognitive impairment. Neurobiol Aging. 2010 Aug;31(8):1443-51, 51 e1.

[18] High-tech scan reveals protein in the brain linked to Alzheimer's disease. A special form of PET scanning offers a more certain diagnosis for some, but at a steep out-of-pocket cost. Harv Mens Health Watch. 2014 Feb;18(7):6.

[19] McKhann G, Drachman D, Folstein M, Katzman R, Price D, Stadlan EM. Clinical diagnosis of Alzheimer's disease: report of the NINCDS-ADRDA Work Group under the auspices of Department of Health and Human Services Task Force on Alzheimer's Disease. Neurology. 1984 Jul;34(7):939-44.

[20] Tanne JH. US scientists discuss early detection and treatment of Alzheimer's disease. BMJ. 2012;344:e1068.

[21] Jack CR, Jr., Knopman DS, Jagust WJ, Shaw LM, Aisen PS, Weiner MW, et al. Hypothetical model of dynamic biomarkers of the Alzheimer's pathological cascade. Lancet Neurol. 2010 Jan;9(1):119-28.

[22] Fjell AM, Walhovd KB. Neuroimaging results impose new views on Alzheimer's disease--the role of amyloid revised. Mol Neurobiol. 2012 Feb;45(1):153-72.

[23] Blennow K. Biomarkers in Alzheimer's disease drug development. Nat Med. 2010 Nov;16(11):1218-22.

[24] Cummings JL. Biomarkers in Alzheimer's disease drug development. Alzheimers Dement. 2011 May;7(3):e13-44.

[25] Hampel H, Blennow K, Shaw LM, Hoessler YC, Zetterberg H, Trojanowski JQ. Total and phosphorylated tau protein as biological markers of Alzheimer's disease. Exp Gerontol. 2010 Jan;45(1):30-40.

[26] de Almeida SM, Shumaker SD, LeBlanc SK, Delaney P, Marquie-Beck J, Ueland S, et al. Incidence of post-dural puncture headache in research volunteers. Headache. 2011 Nov-Dec;51(10):1503-10.

[27] Schoonenboom NS, Mulder C, Vanderstichele H, Van Elk EJ, Kok A, Van Kamp GJ, et al. Effects of processing and storage conditions on amyloid beta (1-42) and tau concentrations in cerebrospinal fluid: implications for use in clinical practice. Clin Chem. 2005 Jan;51(1):189-95.

[28] Kaiser E, Schonknecht P, Thomann PA, Hunt A, Schroder J. Influence of delayed CSF storage on concentrations of phospho-tau protein (181), total tau protein and beta-amyloid (1-42). Neurosci Lett. 2007 May 1;417(2):193-5.

[29] Simonsen AH, Bahl JM, Danborg PB, Lindstrom V, Larsen SO, Grubb A, et al. Pre-analytical factors influencing the stability of cerebrospinal fluid proteins. J Neurosci Methods. 2013 May 15;215(2):234-40.

[30] Morris JC, Blennow K, Froelich L, Nordberg A, Soininen H, Waldemar G, et al. Harmonized diagnostic criteria for Alzheimer's disease: recommendations. J Intern Med. 2014 Mar;275(3):204-13.

[31] Forsberg A, Engler H, Almkvist O, Blomquist G, Hagman G, Wall A, et al. PET imaging of amyloid deposition in patients with mild cognitive impairment. Neurobiol Aging. 2008 Oct;29(10):1456-65.

[32] Yang L, Rieves D, Ganley C. Brain amyloid imaging--FDA approval of florbetapir F18 injection. N Engl J Med. 2012 Sep 6;367(10):885-7.

[33] CMS issues new instructions on PET coverage. J Nucl Med. 2014 Apr;55(4):9N-10N.

[34] Koyama A, Okereke OI, Yang T, Blacker D, Selkoe DJ, Grodstein F. Plasma amyloid-beta as a predictor of dementia and cognitive decline: a systematic review and meta-analysis. Arch Neurol. 2012 Jul;69(7):824-31.

[35] Toledo JB, Shaw LM, Trojanowski JQ. Plasma amyloid beta measurements - a desired but elusive Alzheimer's disease biomarker. Alzheimers Res Ther. 2013;5(2):8.

[36] Mehta PD, Pirttila T, Mehta SP, Sersen EA, Aisen PS, Wisniewski HM. Plasma and cerebrospinal fluid levels of amyloid beta proteins 1-40 and 1-42 in Alzheimer disease. Arch Neurol. 2000 Jan;57(1):100-5.

[37] Perez-Grijalba V, Pesini P, Allue JA, Sarasa L, Montanes M, Lacosta AM, et al. Abeta1-17 is a Major Amyloid-beta Fragment Isoform in Cerebrospinal Fluid and Blood with Possible Diagnostic Value in Alzheimer's Disease. J Alzheimers Dis. 2014 Jul 24.

[38] Wu G, Sankaranarayanan S, Wong J, Tugusheva K, Michener MS, Shi X, et al. Characterization of plasma beta-secretase (BACE1) activity and soluble amyloid precursor proteins as potential biomarkers for Alzheimer's disease. J Neurosci Res. 2012 Dec; 90(12):2247-58.

[39] Kaneko N, Nakamura A, Washimi Y, Kato T, Sakurai T, Arahata Y, et al. Novel plasma biomarker surrogating cerebral amyloid deposition. Proc Jpn Acad Ser B Phys Biol Sci. 2014;90(9):353-64.

[40] Noguchi-Shinohara M, Hamaguchi T, Nozaki I, Sakai K, Yamada M. Serum tau protein as a marker for the diagnosis of Creutzfeldt-Jakob disease. J Neurol. 2011 Aug; 258(8):1464-8.

[41] Blennow K, Hampel H, Weiner M, Zetterberg H. Cerebrospinal fluid and plasma biomarkers in Alzheimer disease. Nat Rev Neurol. 2010 Mar;6(3):131-44.

[42] Neselius S, Zetterberg H, Blennow K, Marcusson J, Brisby H. Increased CSF levels of phosphorylated neurofilament heavy protein following bout in amateur boxers. PLoS One. 2013;8(11):e81249.

[43] Neselius S, Zetterberg H, Blennow K, Randall J, Wilson D, Marcusson J, et al. Olympic boxing is associated with elevated levels of the neuronal protein tau in plasma. Brain Inj. 2013;27(4):425-33.

[44] Randall J, Mortberg E, Provuncher GK, Fournier DR, Duffy DC, Rubertsson S, et al. Tau proteins in serum predict neurological outcome after hypoxic brain injury from cardiac arrest: results of a pilot study. Resuscitation. 2013 Mar;84(3):351-6.

[45] Neumann K, Farias G, Slachevsky A, Perez P, Maccioni RB. Human platelets tau: a potential peripheral marker for Alzheimer's disease. J Alzheimers Dis. 2011;25(1): 103-9.

[46] Upadhaya AR, Lungrin I, Yamaguchi H, Fandrich M, Thal DR. High-molecular weight Abeta oligomers and protofibrils are the predominant Abeta species in the native soluble protein fraction of the AD brain. J Cell Mol Med. 2012 Feb;16(2):287-95.

[47] Yoshiike Y, Chui DH, Akagi T, Tanaka N, Takashima A. Specific compositions of amyloid-beta peptides as the determinant of toxic beta-aggregation. J Biol Chem. 2003 Jun 27;278(26):23648-55.

[48] Savage MJ, Kalinina J, Wolfe A, Tugusheva K, Korn R, Cash-Mason T, et al. A sensitive abeta oligomer assay discriminates Alzheimer's and aged control cerebrospinal fluid. J Neurosci. 2014 Feb 19;34(8):2884-97.

[49] Herskovits AZ, Locascio JJ, Peskind ER, Li G, Hyman BT. A Luminex assay detects amyloid beta oligomers in Alzheimer's disease cerebrospinal fluid. PLoS One. 2013;8(7):e67898.

[50] Kasai T, Tokuda T, Taylor M, Kondo M, Mann DM, Foulds PG, et al. Correlation of Abeta oligomer levels in matched cerebrospinal fluid and serum samples. Neurosci Lett. 2013 Sep 13;551:17-22.

[51] Funke SA. Detection of Soluble Amyloid-beta Oligomers and Insoluble High-Molecular-Weight Particles in CSF: Development of Methods with Potential for Diagnosis and Therapy Monitoring of Alzheimer's Disease. Int J Alzheimers Dis. 2011;2011:151645.

[52] Yang T, Hong S, O'Malley T, Sperling RA, Walsh DM, Selkoe DJ. New ELISAs with high specificity for soluble oligomers of amyloid beta-protein detect natural Abeta oligomers in human brain but not CSF. Alzheimers Dement. 2013 Mar;9(2):99-112.

[53] Zhang J, Peng M, Jia J. Plasma Amyloid-beta Oligomers and Soluble Tumor Necrosis Factor Receptors as Potential Biomarkers of AD. Curr Alzheimer Res. 2014 Mar 16.

[54] Kiddle SJ, Sattlecker M, Proitsi P, Simmons A, Westman E, Bazenet C, et al. Candidate blood proteome markers of Alzheimer's disease onset and progression: a systematic review and replication study. J Alzheimers Dis. 2014;38(3):515-31.

[55] O'Bryant SE, Xiao G, Barber R, Reisch J, Doody R, Fairchild T, et al. A serum protein-based algorithm for the detection of Alzheimer disease. Arch Neurol. 2010 Sep;67(9): 1077-81.

[56] O'Bryant SE, Xiao G, Barber R, Reisch J, Hall J, Cullum CM, et al. A blood-based algorithm for the detection of Alzheimer's disease. Dement Geriatr Cogn Disord. 2011;32(1):55-62.

[57] Ray S, Britschgi M, Herbert C, Takeda-Uchimura Y, Boxer A, Blennow K, et al. Classification and prediction of clinical Alzheimer's diagnosis based on plasma signaling proteins. Nat Med. 2007 Nov;13(11):1359-62.

[58] Soares HD, Chen Y, Sabbagh M, Roher A, Schrijvers E, Breteler M. Identifying early markers of Alzheimer's disease using quantitative multiplex proteomic immunoassay panels. Ann N Y Acad Sci. 2009 Oct;1180:56-67.

[59] Laske C, Leyhe T, Stransky E, Hoffmann N, Fallgatter AJ, Dietzsch J. Identification of a blood-based biomarker panel for classification of Alzheimer's disease. Int J Neuropsychopharmacol. 2011 Oct;14(9):1147-55.

[60] O'Brien D LS, Kuhn K, Shulz-Knappe P, Ward M,Byers H, Pike I, editor. Tandem mass tags and MRM mass spectrometry for the evaluation of biomarkers implicated in Alzheimer's disease. MP309 Proceedings of the 56th American Society of MAss Spectrometry conference Denver, CO; 2008.

[61] Di Paolo G, Kim TW. Linking lipids to Alzheimer's disease: cholesterol and beyond. Nat Rev Neurosci. 2011 May;12(5):284-96.

[62] Mapstone M, Cheema AK, Fiandaca MS, Zhong X, Mhyre TR, MacArthur LH, et al. Plasma phospholipids identify antecedent memory impairment in older adults. Nat Med. 2014 Apr;20(4):415-8.

[63] Han X, Rozen S, Boyle SH, Hellegers C, Cheng H, Burke JR, et al. Metabolomics in early Alzheimer's disease: identification of altered plasma sphingolipidome using shotgun lipidomics. PLoS One. 2011;6(7):e21643.

[64] Mielke MM, Haughey NJ, Bandaru VV, Weinberg DD, Darby E, Zaidi N, et al. Plasma sphingomyelins are associated with cognitive progression in Alzheimer's disease. J Alzheimers Dis. 2011;27(2):259-69.

[65] Oresic M, Hyotylainen T, Herukka SK, Sysi-Aho M, Mattila I, Seppanan-Laakso T, et al. Metabolome in progression to Alzheimer's disease. Transl Psychiatry. 2011;1:e57.

[66] Spann NJ, Garmire LX, McDonald JG, Myers DS, Milne SB, Shibata N, et al. Regulated accumulation of desmosterol integrates macrophage lipid metabolism and inflammatory responses. Cell. 2012 Sep 28;151(1):138-52.

[67] Hu X, Wang Y, Hao LY, Liu X, Lesch CA, Sanchez BM, et al. Sterol metabolism controls T(H)17 differentiation by generating endogenous RORgamma agonists. Nat Chem Biol. 2015 Feb;11(2):141-7.

[68] Sato Y, Suzuki I, Nakamura T, Bernier F, Aoshima K, Oda Y. Identification of a new plasma biomarker of Alzheimer's disease using metabolomics technology. J Lipid Res. 2012 Mar;53(3):567-76.

[69] Jansen LA. Ethical concerns relating to the detection and treatment of ovarian cancer. Gynecol Oncol. 2002 Jan;84(1):1-3.

[70] Jansen M, Wang W, Greco D, Bellenchi GC, di Porzio U, Brown AJ, et al. What dictates the accumulation of desmosterol in the developing brain? FASEB J. 2013 Mar; 27(3):865-70.

[71] Vance JE. Dysregulation of cholesterol balance in the brain: contribution to neurodegenerative diseases. Dis Model Mech. 2012 Nov;5(6):746-55.

[72] Karasinska JM, Hayden MR. Cholesterol metabolism in Huntington disease. Nat Rev Neurol. 2011 Oct;7(10):561-72.

[73] Popp J, Meichsner S, Kolsch H, Lewczuk P, Maier W, Kornhuber J, et al. Cerebral and extracerebral cholesterol metabolism and CSF markers of Alzheimer's disease. Biochem Pharmacol. 2013 Jul 1;86(1):37-42.

[74] Sato Y, Bernier F, Yamanaka Y, Aoshima K, Oda Y, Ingelsson M, et al. Reduced plasma desmosterol/cholesterol and longitudinal cognitive decline in Alzheimer's dis-

ease. Alzheimer's & Dementia: Diagnosis, Assessment & Disease Monitoring. 2014; (in press).

[75] Swaminathan S, Shen L, Risacher SL, Yoder KK, West JD, Kim S, et al. Amyloid pathway-based candidate gene analysis of [(11)C]PiB-PET in the Alzheimer's Disease Neuroimaging Initiative (ADNI) cohort. Brain Imaging Behav. 2012 Mar;6(1):1-15.

[76] Booij BB, Lindahl T, Wetterberg P, Skaane NV, Saebo S, Feten G, et al. A gene expression pattern in blood for the early detection of Alzheimer's disease. J Alzheimers Dis. 2011;23(1):109-19.

[77] Fehlbaum-Beurdeley P, Sol O, Desire L, Touchon J, Dantoine T, Vercelletto M, et al. Validation of AclarusDx, a blood-based transcriptomic signature for the diagnosis of Alzheimer's disease. J Alzheimers Dis. 2012;32(1):169-81.

[78] Lunnon K, Sattlecker M, Furney SJ, Coppola G, Simmons A, Proitsi P, et al. A blood gene expression marker of early Alzheimer's disease. J Alzheimers Dis. 2013;33(3): 737-53.

[79] Lunnon K, Ibrahim Z, Proitsi P, Lourdusamy A, Newhouse S, Sattlecker M, et al. Mitochondrial dysfunction and immune activation are detectable in early Alzheimer's disease blood. J Alzheimers Dis. 2012;30(3):685-710.

[80] Chong MS, Goh LK, Lim WS, Chan M, Tay L, Chen G, et al. Gene expression profiling of peripheral blood leukocytes shows consistent longitudinal downregulation of TOMM40 and upregulation of KIR2DL5A, PLOD1, and SLC2A8 among fast progressors in early Alzheimer's disease. J Alzheimers Dis. 2013;34(2):399-405.

[81] Zampetaki A, Willeit P, Drozdov I, Kiechl S, Mayr M. Profiling of circulating microRNAs: from single biomarkers to re-wired networks. Cardiovasc Res. 2012 Mar 15;93(4):555-62.

[82] Guo H, Ingolia NT, Weissman JS, Bartel DP. Mammalian microRNAs predominantly act to decrease target mRNA levels. Nature. 2010 Aug 12;466(7308):835-40.

[83] Filipowicz W, Bhattacharyya SN, Sonenberg N. Mechanisms of post-transcriptional regulation by microRNAs: are the answers in sight? Nat Rev Genet. 2008 Feb;9(2): 102-14.

[84] Lu M, Zhang Q, Deng M, Miao J, Guo Y, Gao W, et al. An analysis of human microRNA and disease associations. PLoS One. 2008;3(10):e3420.

[85] Esquela-Kerscher A, Slack FJ. Oncomirs - microRNAs with a role in cancer. Nat Rev Cancer. 2006 Apr;6(4):259-69.

[86] Vickers KC, Palmisano BT, Shoucri BM, Shamburek RD, Remaley AT. MicroRNAs are transported in plasma and delivered to recipient cells by high-density lipoproteins. Nat Cell Biol. 2011 Apr;13(4):423-33.

[87] Gallo A, Tandon M, Alevizos I, Illei GG. The majority of microRNAs detectable in serum and saliva is concentrated in exosomes. PLoS One. 2012;7(3):e30679.

[88] Michael A, Bajracharya SD, Yuen PS, Zhou H, Star RA, Illei GG, et al. Exosomes from human saliva as a source of microRNA biomarkers. Oral Dis. 2010 Jan;16(1):34-8.

[89] Wang D, Qiu C, Zhang H, Wang J, Cui Q, Yin Y. Human microRNA oncogenes and tumor suppressors show significantly different biological patterns: from functions to targets. PLoS One. 2010;5(9).

[90] Arroyo JD, Chevillet JR, Kroh EM, Ruf IK, Pritchard CC, Gibson DF, et al. Argonaute2 complexes carry a population of circulating microRNAs independent of vesicles in human plasma. Proc Natl Acad Sci U S A. 2011 Mar 22;108(12):5003-8.

[91] Turchinovich A, Weiz L, Langheinz A, Burwinkel B. Characterization of extracellular circulating microRNA. Nucleic Acids Res. 2011 Sep 1;39(16):7223-33.

[92] Xu J, Wu C, Che X, Wang L, Yu D, Zhang T, et al. Circulating microRNAs, miR-21, miR-122, and miR-223, in patients with hepatocellular carcinoma or chronic hepatitis. Mol Carcinog. 2011 Feb;50(2):136-42.

[93] Roth P, Wischhusen J, Happold C, Chandran PA, Hofer S, Eisele G, et al. A specific miRNA signature in the peripheral blood of glioblastoma patients. J Neurochem. 2011 Aug;118(3):449-57.

[94] Malumbres R, Sarosiek KA, Cubedo E, Ruiz JW, Jiang X, Gascoyne RD, et al. Differentiation stage-specific expression of microRNAs in B lymphocytes and diffuse large B-cell lymphomas. Blood. 2009 Apr 16;113(16):3754-64.

[95] Dong Y, Wu WK, Wu CW, Sung JJ, Yu J, Ng SS. MicroRNA dysregulation in colorectal cancer: a clinical perspective. Br J Cancer. 2011 Mar 15;104(6):893-8.

[96] Li J, Wang Y, Yu W, Chen J, Luo J. Expression of serum miR-221 in human hepatocellular carcinoma and its prognostic significance. Biochem Biophys Res Commun. 2011 Mar 4;406(1):70-3.

[97] Delay C, Hebert SS. MicroRNAs and Alzheimer's Disease Mouse Models: Current Insights and Future Research Avenues. Int J Alzheimers Dis. 2011;2011:894938.

[98] Long JM, Ray B, Lahiri DK. MicroRNA-153 physiologically inhibits expression of amyloid-beta precursor protein in cultured human fetal brain cells and is dysregulated in a subset of Alzheimer disease patients. J Biol Chem. 2012 Sep 7;287(37): 31298-310.

[99] Long JM, Lahiri DK. MicroRNA-101 downregulates Alzheimer's amyloid-beta precursor protein levels in human cell cultures and is differentially expressed. Biochem Biophys Res Commun. 2011 Jan 28;404(4):889-95.

[100] John B, Enright AJ, Aravin A, Tuschl T, Sander C, Marks DS. Human MicroRNA targets. PLoS Biol. 2004 Nov;2(11):e363.

[101] Patel N, Hoang D, Miller N, Ansaloni S, Huang Q, Rogers JT, et al. MicroRNAs can regulate human APP levels. Mol Neurodegener. 2008;3:10.

[102] Hebert SS, Horre K, Nicolai L, Papadopoulou AS, Mandemakers W, Silahtaroglu AN, et al. Loss of microRNA cluster miR-29a/b-1 in sporadic Alzheimer's disease correlates with increased BACE1/beta-secretase expression. Proc Natl Acad Sci U S A. 2008 Apr 29;105(17):6415-20.

[103] Geekiyanage H, Jicha GA, Nelson PT, Chan C. Blood serum miRNA: non-invasive biomarkers for Alzheimer's disease. Exp Neurol. 2012 Jun;235(2):491-6.

[104] Mizuno H, Nakamura A, Aoki Y, Ito N, Kishi S, Yamamoto K, et al. Identification of muscle-specific microRNAs in serum of muscular dystrophy animal models: promising novel blood-based markers for muscular dystrophy. PLoS One. 2011;6(3):e18388.

[105] Cuk K, Zucknick M, Heil J, Madhavan D, Schott S, Turchinovich A, et al. Circulating microRNAs in plasma as early detection markers for breast cancer. Int J Cancer. 2013 Apr 1;132(7):1602-12.

[106] Schipper HM, Maes OC, Chertkow HM, Wang E. MicroRNA expression in Alzheimer blood mononuclear cells. Gene Regul Syst Bio. 2007;1:263-74.

[107] Cogswell JP, Ward J, Taylor IA, Waters M, Shi Y, Cannon B, et al. Identification of miRNA changes in Alzheimer's disease brain and CSF yields putative biomarkers and insights into disease pathways. J Alzheimers Dis. 2008 May;14(1):27-41.

[108] Kumar P, Dezso Z, MacKenzie C, Oestreicher J, Agoulnik S, Byrne M, et al. Circulating miRNA biomarkers for Alzheimer's disease. PLoS One. 2013;8(7):e69807.

[109] Lin L, Lesnick TG, Maraganore DM, Isacson O. Axon guidance and synaptic maintenance: preclinical markers for neurodegenerative disease and therapeutics. Trends Neurosci. 2009 Mar;32(3):142-9.

[110] Gallo G. Tau is actin up in Alzheimer's disease. Nat Cell Biol. 2007 Feb;9(2):133-4.

[111] Wu F, Yao PJ. Clathrin-mediated endocytosis and Alzheimer's disease: an update. Ageing Res Rev. 2009 Jul;8(3):147-9.

[112] Chacon PJ, Garcia-Mejias R, Rodriguez-Tebar A. Inhibition of RhoA GTPase and the subsequent activation of PTP1B protects cultured hippocampal neurons against amyloid beta toxicity. Mol Neurodegener. 2011;6(1):14.

[113] Saunders AM, Strittmatter WJ, Schmechel D, George-Hyslop PH, Pericak-Vance MA, Joo SH, et al. Association of apolipoprotein E allele epsilon 4 with late-onset familial and sporadic Alzheimer's disease. Neurology. 1993 Aug;43(8):1467-72.

[114] Harold D, Abraham R, Hollingworth P, Sims R, Gerrish A, Hamshere ML, et al. Genome-wide association study identifies variants at CLU and PICALM associated with Alzheimer's disease. Nat Genet. 2009 Oct;41(10):1088-93.

[115] Hollingworth P, Harold D, Sims R, Gerrish A, Lambert JC, Carrasquillo MM, et al. Common variants at ABCA7, MS4A6A/MS4A4E, EPHA1, CD33 and CD2AP are associated with Alzheimer's disease. Nat Genet. 2011 May;43(5):429-35.

[116] McGuinness B, Passmore P. Can statins prevent or help treat Alzheimer's disease? J Alzheimers Dis. 2010;20(3):925-33.

[117] Tan L, Yu JT, Tan MS, Liu QY, Wang HF, Zhang W, et al. Genome-wide serum microRNA expression profiling identifies serum biomarkers for Alzheimer's disease. J Alzheimers Dis. 2014;40(4):1017-27.

[118] McDermott AM, Kerin MJ, Miller N. Identification and validation of miRNAs as endogenous controls for RQ-PCR in blood specimens for breast cancer studies. PLoS One. 2013;8(12):e83718.

[119] Chen ZH, Zhang GL, Li HR, Luo JD, Li ZX, Chen GM, et al. A panel of five circulating microRNAs as potential biomarkers for prostate cancer. Prostate. 2012 Sep 15;72(13):1443-52.

[120] Dickerson BC, Wolk DA. Biomarker-based prediction of progression in MCI: Comparison of AD signature and hippocampal volume with spinal fluid amyloid-beta and tau. Front Aging Neurosci. 2013;5:55.

[121] Leidinger P, Backes C, Deutscher S, Schmitt K, Mueller SC, Frese K, et al. A blood based 12-miRNA signature of Alzheimer disease patients. Genome Biol. 2013;14(7):R78.

[122] Galimberti D, Villa C, Fenoglio C, Serpente M, Ghezzi L, Cioffi SM, et al. Circulating miRNAs as Potential Biomarkers in Alzheimer's Disease. J Alzheimers Dis. 2014 Jul 7.

[123] Jarry J, Schadendorf D, Greenwood C, Spatz A, van Kempen LC. The validity of circulating microRNAs in oncology: five years of challenges and contradictions. Mol Oncol. 2014 Jun;8(4):819-29.

[124] Kim YK, Yeo J, Kim B, Ha M, Kim VN. Short structured RNAs with low GC content are selectively lost during extraction from a small number of cells. Mol Cell. 2012 Jun 29;46(6):893-5.

[125] Zhang X, Azhar G, Wei JY. The expression of microRNA and microRNA clusters in the aging heart. PLoS One. 2012;7(4):e34688.

[126] Kirschner MB, Edelman JJ, Kao SC, Vallely MP, van Zandwijk N, Reid G. The Impact of Hemolysis on Cell-Free microRNA Biomarkers. Front Genet. 2013;4:94.

[127] Blondal T, Jensby Nielsen S, Baker A, Andreasen D, Mouritzen P, Wrang Teilum M, et al. Assessing sample and miRNA profile quality in serum and plasma or other biofluids. Methods. 2013 Jan;59(1):S1-6.

[128] Cheng HH, Yi HS, Kim Y, Kroh EM, Chien JW, Eaton KD, et al. Plasma processing conditions substantially influence circulating microRNA biomarker levels. PLoS One. 2013;8(6):e64795.

[129] Leshkowitz D, Horn-Saban S, Parmet Y, Feldmesser E. Differences in microRNA detection levels are technology and sequence dependent. RNA. 2013 Apr;19(4):527-38.

[130] Yin S, Ho CK, Shuman S. Structure-function analysis of T4 RNA ligase 2. J Biol Chem. 2003 May 16;278(20):17601-8.

[131] Mestdagh P, Hartmann N, Baeriswyl L, Andreasen D, Bernard N, Chen C, et al. Evaluation of quantitative miRNA expression platforms in the microRNA quality control (miRQC) study. Nat Methods. 2014 Aug;11(8):809-15.

[132] Meyer SU, Pfaffl MW, Ulbrich SE. Normalization strategies for microRNA profiling experiments: a 'normal' way to a hidden layer of complexity? Biotechnol Lett. 2010 Dec;32(12):1777-88.

[133] Pradervand S, Weber J, Thomas J, Bueno M, Wirapati P, Lefort K, et al. Impact of normalization on miRNA microarray expression profiling. RNA. 2009 Mar;15(3):493-501.

[134] Ikram MK, Cheung CY, Wong TY, Chen CP. Retinal pathology as biomarker for cognitive impairment and Alzheimer's disease. J Neurol Neurosurg Psychiatry. 2012 Sep;83(9):917-22.

[135] Chen Y, Shi S, Zhang J, Gao H, Liu H, Wang J, et al. [Diagnostic value of AD7C-NTP for patients with mild cognitive impairment due to Alzheimer's disease]. Zhonghua Yi Xue Za Zhi. 2014 Jun 3;94(21):1613-7.

[136] Youn YC, Park KW, Han SH, Kim S. Urine neural thread protein measurements in Alzheimer disease. J Am Med Dir Assoc. 2011 Jun;12(5):372-6.

[137] Ma L, Chen J, Wang R, Han Y, Zhang J, Dong W, et al. Alzheimer-associated urine neuronal thread protein level increases with age in a healthy Chinese population. J Clin Neurosci. 2014 Aug 21.

[138] Watt AD, Perez KA, Rembach AR, Masters CL, Villemagne VL, Barnham KJ. Variability in blood-based amyloid-beta assays: the need for consensus on pre-analytical processing. J Alzheimers Dis. 2012;30(2):323-36.

[139] Thambisetty M, Lovestone S. Blood-based biomarkers of Alzheimer's disease: challenging but feasible. Biomark Med. 2010 Feb;4(1):65-79.

[140] Josephs KA, Petersen RC, Knopman DS, Boeve BF, Whitwell JL, Duffy JR, et al. Clinicopathologic analysis of frontotemporal and corticobasal degenerations and PSP. Neurology. 2006 Jan 10;66(1):41-8.

[141] Norton MC, Smith KR, Ostbye T, Tschanz JT, Corcoran C, Schwartz S, et al. Greater risk of dementia when spouse has dementia? The Cache County study. J Am Geriatr Soc. 2010 May;58(5):895-900.

[142] Honjo K, van Reekum R, Verhoeff NP. Alzheimer's disease and infection: do infectious agents contribute to progression of Alzheimer's disease? Alzheimers Dement. 2009 Jul;5(4):348-60.

[143] Itzhaki RF, Wozniak MA, Appelt DM, Balin BJ. Infiltration of the brain by pathogens causes Alzheimer's disease. Neurobiol Aging. 2004 May-Jun;25(5):619-27.

5

Neuroinflammation and Alteration of the Blood-Brain Barrier in Alzheimer´s Disease

Luis Oskar Soto-Rojas, Fidel de la Cruz-López,
Miguel Angel Ontiveros Torres,
Amparo Viramontes-Pintos,
María del Carmen Cárdenas-Aguayo,
Marco A. Meraz-Ríos, Citlaltepetl Salinas-Lara,
Benjamín Florán-Garduño and José Luna-Muñoz

1. Introduction

Alzheimer's disease (AD) is a neurodegenerative disease, characterized by progressive memory loss, cognitive deterioration and personality changes. Neuropathologically AD brains are characterized by massive accumulation of neurofibrillary tangles (NFT). NFTs are composed by paired helical filaments (PHF), which main constituent is tau protein. Another hallmark lesions of AD are Neuritic plaques (NPs), constituted by extracellular amyloid peptide aggregates (Aβ), that are associated with distrophyc neurites (DNs). Amyloid precursor protein (APP) processing occurs via two pathways. A) The amyloidogenic and B) the non-amyloidogenic pathway. In the amyloidogenic pathway, the APP is proteolyzed by β-secretase. This truncation occurs at the N-terminus of APP. The cleavage produces a soluble N-terminal fragment of APP (sAPPβ) and a C-terminal transmembrane fragment (β-CTF). β-CTF is cut into the membrane by γ-secretase and generates the Amyloid beta (Aβ) peptide and the APP intracellular domain (AICD). Depending on the site of γ-secretase cleavage, two main species of Aβ are generated: Aβ 40 and Aβ 42 amino acids. Aβ 42 is more hydrophobic and more prone to aggregate, as compared to the Aβ 40 peptide. In the non-amyloidogenic pathway, APP is cleaved by the α-secretase. This cleavage occurs in the middle region of Aβ and produces an N-terminal fragment of soluble APPα (sAPPα) and a C-terminal transmembrane (α-CTF) fragment. The sAPPα have neurotrophic and neuroprotective functions.

Similarly to β-CTF, α-CTF after being cleaved by γ-secretase generates a 23-25 amino acid peptide designated as p3. Aβ aggregates promote an inflammatory response mediated by activated microglia and astrocytes, that may activate pathological signalling pathways, leading to neurodegeneration. Long-term activation of the innate immune system is able to trigger an inflammatory cascade that converges on alterations of the cytoskeleton (including aggregation of tau protein and formation of PHFs and microtube disassembling) promoting neuronal degeneration. One of the pathological signalling pathways that may lead to neurodegeneration is oxidative stress, defined by the generation of a large amount of reactive oxygen species (ROS), which are highly harmful since they lead to the alteration in the structure of proteins, lipids and nucleic acids and cellular death. High levels of copper and iron have been detected in the blood plasma of people with AD. These metals catalyse the production of ROS by the Fenton reaction resulting in the generation of highly reactive hydroxyl radical, so that the reactivity of these metals can give rise to cellular damage and neurodegeneration. In AD, it had been described oxidative stress caused by free radicals (FRs). The most important in human biology FRs are superoxide (O_2 -), hydroxyl ($OH\cdot$), nitric oxide ($NO\cdot$), and trichloro-methyl ($CCl_3\cdot$). In AD, there is an increase in iron concentration in the hippocampus. There is an accumulation of iron and aluminum in NPs and cerebrospinal fluid (CSF), which could contribute to this oxidative stress. In AD, neuroinflammation is involved in multiple patho-logical mechanisms. Clinicopathological and neuroimaging studies have shown that inflam-mation and microglial activation precede neuronal damage and that oxidative stress occurs prior to neurodegeneration. Aβ accumulation alters the normal neuronal function, cell death, even before the formation of NPs and NFTs. Aβ not only has been linked to the inflammatory response, but also in a lesser extent to tau pathology. The Aβ itself causes activation of microglia and astrocytes through toll-like receptors 2, 4, 9 (TLR); activated microglia produces neurotoxic molecules and is conveniently located to the vicinity of the NPs. The proinflam-matory cascade generated by microglial activation, results in the release of cytotoxic molecules such cytokines, chemokines, matrix metalloproteinases, and complement factors. These cytotoxic molecules may enhance neuronal neurodegeneration increasing sensitivity to FRs. The neurotoxicity mediated by microglial cells depends on ROS and cytokines. The present chapter address the physiological and pathological role of proinflammatory cytokines and the induction of tau pathology including tau accumulation and the formation of NFTs, as well as the mechanisms involving extracellular deposits of beta amyloid species (Aβ1-42, Aβ1-40, Aβ3-42 and Aβ11-42), which generate neurotoxic microenvironment in AD. In relation with the mechanisms involved in AD neuroinflammation, we will discuss the participation of caspases in inflammation and its likely activation as a result of the accumulation of endothelial cells. We will also talk about how the accumulation of Aβ in blood vessels affects blood-brain barrier endothelial cells tight junctions, modifying its permeability and its implications in AD pathology.

2. Diagnosis of Alzheimer's disease

AD can be diagnosed with 70% of accuracy, with a battery of clinical analysis and cognition tests. However, the definitive diagnostic test for AD is done post-mortem through histological analysis of the brains of patients.

2.1. Gross microscopy pathology

Atrophy of the brain in a case of AD, is generally symmetrical and diffuse in the convolutions, which is evidenced by the decrease in thickness. An increase in the depth of the grooves, a dilatation of the ventricles (Fig 1A and B compared to Fig 1 C and D) and decreased brain weight and volume is noticeable. Atrophy, mainly affecting the hippocampus, and the adjacent area transenthorinal, entorhinal cortex and the temporal and frontal lobes (Fig 1 C,D).

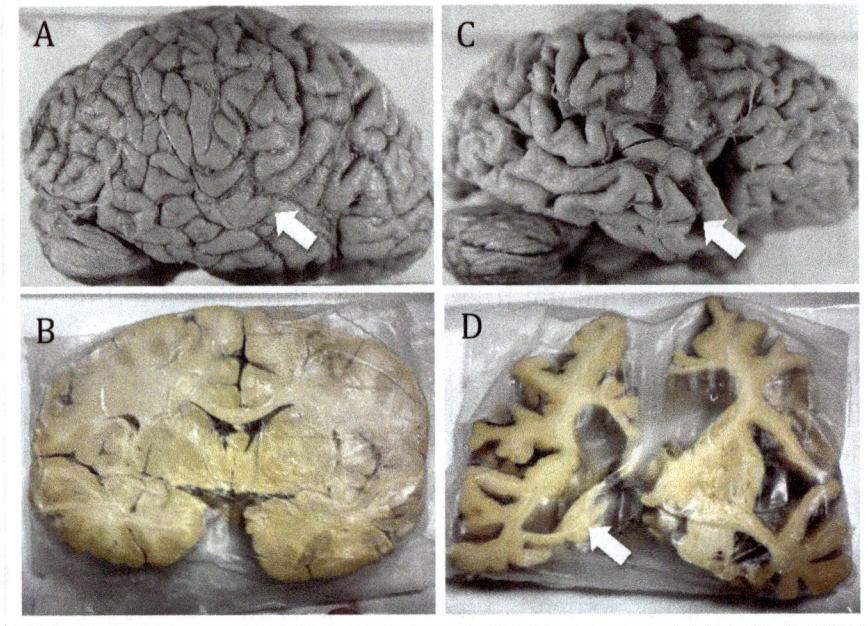

Figure 1. Neuroanatomical comparison of normal brain and Alzheimer's disease brain. A,B) Normal Brain. C,D) Brain with pathology of AD. B) Prominent atrophy seen in fronto-temporal areas involved with association functions (arrows). B, D) Coronal sections of A) and C) respectively. Where observe an enlargement of the ventricles and selective hippocampal atrophy (arrow).

2.2. Histopathology of Alzheimer's disease

Microscopically, AD is characterized by the presence of lesions in the brain tissue known as neurofibrillary tangles (NFTs. Fig. 2 A, B. long arrows), dystrophic neurites (DNs. Fig. 1 C short arrows) and neuritic plaques (NPs, Fig. 1. C).

2.3. Neurofibrillary tangles

It has been shown that the severity of dementia in AD, correlates significantly with the density of NFTs in the neocortex and entorhinal cortex [1, 2]. At the stage of degeneration NFTs may be intracellular (iNFT, Fig. 2A) or extracellular (eNFT, Fig. 2B), [3] The formation of NFTs is associated with neuronal death [4-6] and found a strong correlation between neuronal degeneration and the transition between iNFT and eNFT [7]. The iNFT are characterized by a compact consistency and to be able to distinguish the cell membrane and the nucleus, although the nucleus may be displaced from its original position by the inclusion of fibrils. NFT is such a typical flame shape (Fig.2A). The eNFT show a fibrillar relax form and without nucleus (Fig 2B). These eNFT, are considered as the "skeleton" or "ghost" of the affected neuron (Fig 2B), are released into the extracellular space as a consequence of cell death, which remain stable due to its high insolubility and resistance to proteolysis.

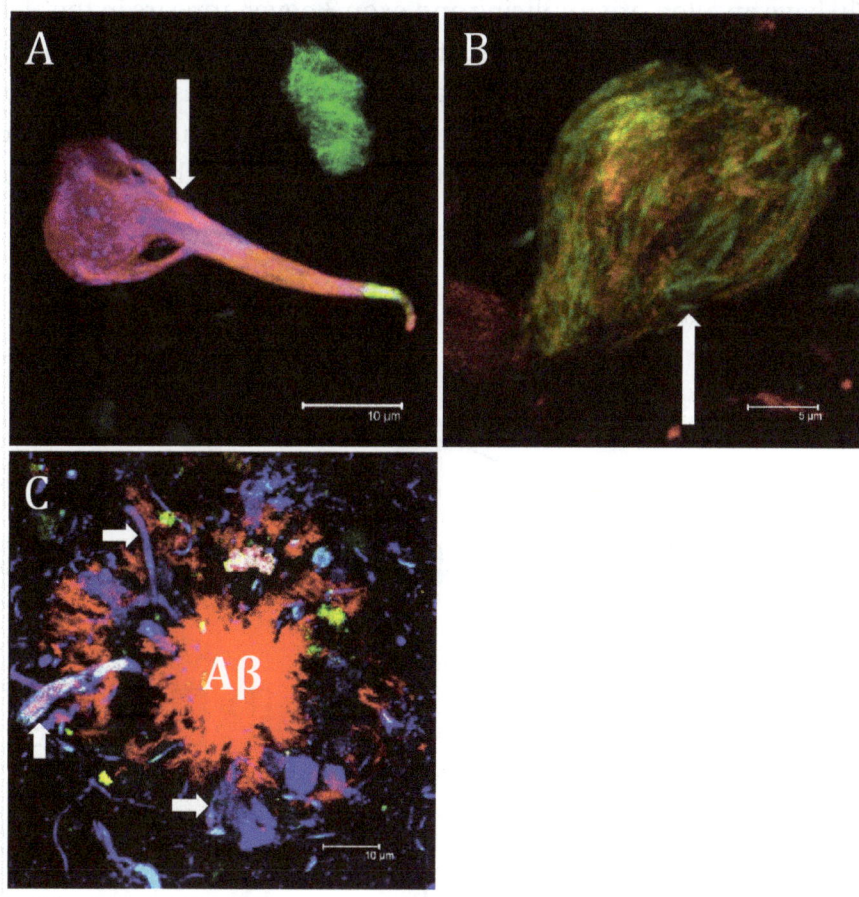

Figure 2. Hallmark characteristic of Alzheimer's disease brains. A) intracellular neurofibrillary tangle B) extracellular neurofibrillary tangle, are evidenced with antibodies against protein tau. C) Neuritic plaque. Evidenced by thiazine red dye (red channel) marker of beta-pleated sheet conformation and doble immunolabelling with two antibodies raised against tau protein to evidence dystrophic neurites (arrows), associated with these beta amyloid deposits (Aβ). Confocal microscope images (Leica SP8).

3. The tau protein and paired helical filaments

The NTFs and DNs (a component of NPs) are formed by the accumulation of abnormal polymers know as paired helical filaments (PHFs), due to their ultrastructural appearance [8]. The PHFs are characterized by its staining with thiazine red fluorescent dye, which has affinity for β-pleated structures [9], and have been used to differentiate between non-fibrillar (pre-assembled) amorphous and fibrillar states (assembled) of tau protein in AD [3, 10]. The main structural constituent of PHFs is tau protein, which is normally associated with microtubules.

3.1. Tau protein structure

Tau is the major component of the family of microtubule-associated proteins in the neuron. The tau gene was located on the long arm of chromosome 17 (17q21) and contains 16 exons[11]. Three of these exons (exon 4, 6 and 8), occurs only in the peripheral tissue RNA and these are not present in human brain mRNA, exons 1 and 14 are transcribed but not translated [12-15]. Exons 2, 3 and 10 have an alternative splicing and exon 3 never appears in the absence of exon 2 [15, 16]. Alternative splicing of three exons latter produces six isoforms of tau protein in the adult brain [12, 17]. Tau isoforms differ from each other by the presence or absence of one or two inserts (29 or 58 amino acids) in the amino terminal portion and by the presence of 3 to 4 repeated domains in the carboxyl terminal portion. The length of the various isoforms of tau varies from 352-441 aa's (Fig 3) [18].

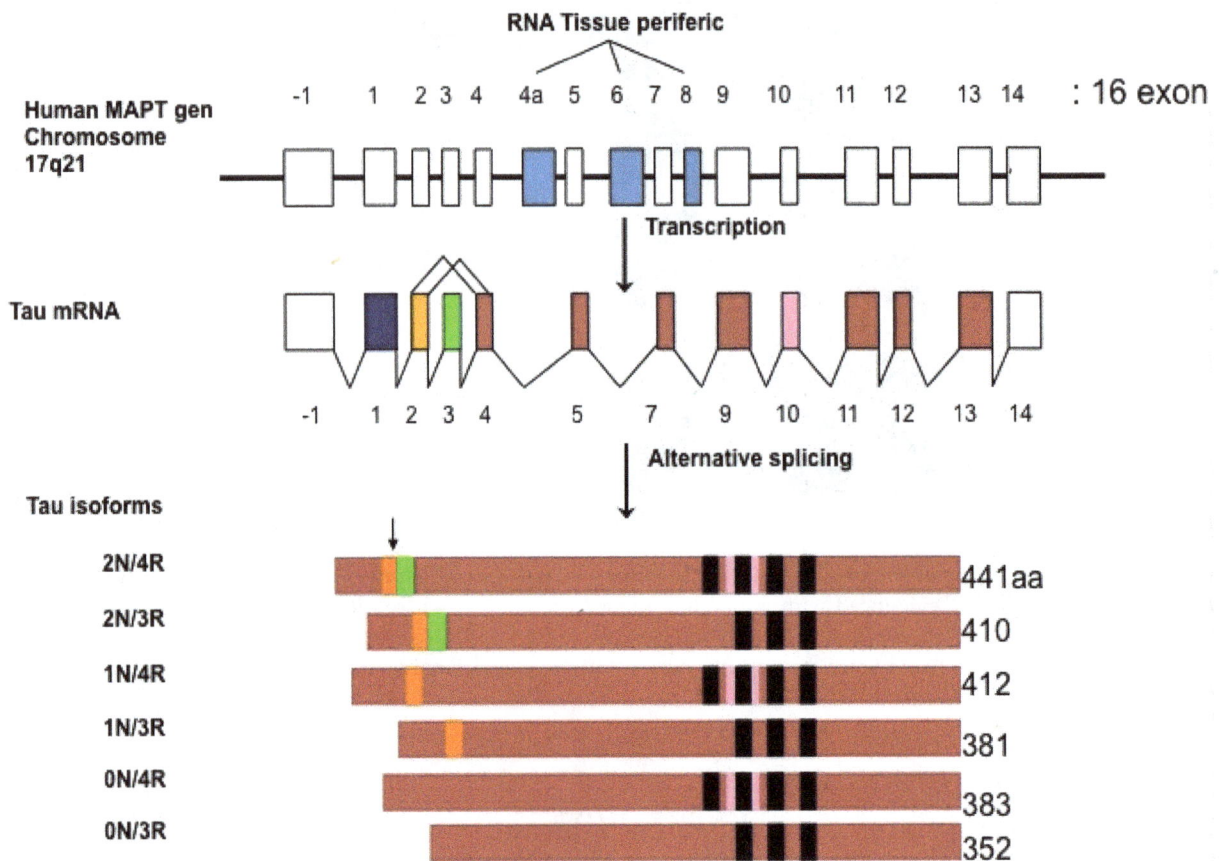

Figure 3. Schematic representation of tau protein gene. The MAPT gene encoding the tau protein is located on chromosome 17q21, which contains 16 exons. Isoforms of tau protein in human brain is encoded by 11 exons. Exons 2, 3 and 10 are alternatively spliced, favouring the synthesis of 6 isoforms. With a range of longitude between 352-441 amino acids. They differ by the presence or absence of one or two inserts of 29 amino acids at its amino terminal portion and by the presence of 3 or 4 microtubule binding domains in its C-terminal portion.

3.2. Post-translational modifications of tau protein in AD

It has not been reported for AD any change in the levels of RNAs messenger of any of the existing six isoforms of tau protein, which suggested, from the beginning, that abnormal forms of the protein found in PHFs originate from posttranslational modification rather than the novo synthesis [12]. There are two posttranslational modifications of tau protein, as the major molecular mechanisms involved in the pathophysiology of AD: the abnormal hyperphosphorylation and endogenous proteolysis [19, 20]. Both pathological processes are involved in the cascade of molecular events that lead to irreversible polymerization of tau protein into PHFs. Recently it has been described a series of tau conformational changes which appear to be associated, in fact, they appear to be the consequence of both the endogenous hyperphosphorylation and the truncation [21, 22].

4. Neuritic plaques

NPs are composed of extracellular deposits of insoluble amyloid fibrils that are made-up of Aβ peptide (Fig 2C), and these deposits are associated with neuritic component from dendritic and axonal origin (Fig. 2B arrows). There could also be AD brains with soluble non-fibrillar β-amyloid deposits without DNs associated, named senile plaques (SPs). SPs do not have a selective topographic distribution, however, their density is predominant in motor or sensory cortical areas than in primary hippocampal. The density of NPs in AD, in general, does not have a good correlation with the progression of dementia and the degree of neuronal loss [5, 23].

5. Amyloid precursor protein and amyloid-β peptide

Aβ originates from a large trans-membrane molecule, called APP. So far 8 isoforms of APP are known, were the predominats are the ones of 695, 751 and 770 aa's. The 695 isoform is the most abundant neuronal isoform. APP is a membrane glycoprotein with a single transmembrane domain, an intracytoplasmic portion and a extracellular long portion (Fig. 4). APP has an hydrophobic region of 23 aa's, by which it is anchored to cell membrane. The extracellular domain exposed to partial proteolysis by the action of three secretases (α, β and γ) (Fig 4). The proteolytic processing of APP, can occur via two types: the amyloidogenic and the non-amyloidogenic. By the action of both enzymes: γ (presenilin 1) [24] and β (transmembrane aspartyl protease called BACE) secretases, fragments of Aβ are generated, predominantly the fragments of 40 and 42 aa's. Alternatively to this proteolytic pathway amyloidogenic form, the action of α-secretase (metallo-protease and call disintegrin TACE) that cleaves the sequence of Aβ at aa's 16 and 17, represents a non-amyloidogenic processing. At first it was thought that the Aβ was produced only in pathological events, however, it was demonstrated that its production and secretion are physiological process, and Aβ is present in plasma and cerebro-spinal fluid during the normal life of an individual [9, 25, 26]. In AD, APP metabolism is altered with a progressive increase in the production and abnormal deposition of Aβ. There are some Aβ deposits without neuritic component in elderly individuals without cognitive impairment

[27]. In general, it is thought that the abnormal accumulation of Aβ may be depend on certain alterations in the normal metabolic APP processes. Recent studies have emphasized a neuro-toxic role of Aβ in *in vivo* animals models, which have led to reconsider the Aβ peptide, as one of the main factors related to the molecular pathogenesis of AD [28-30].

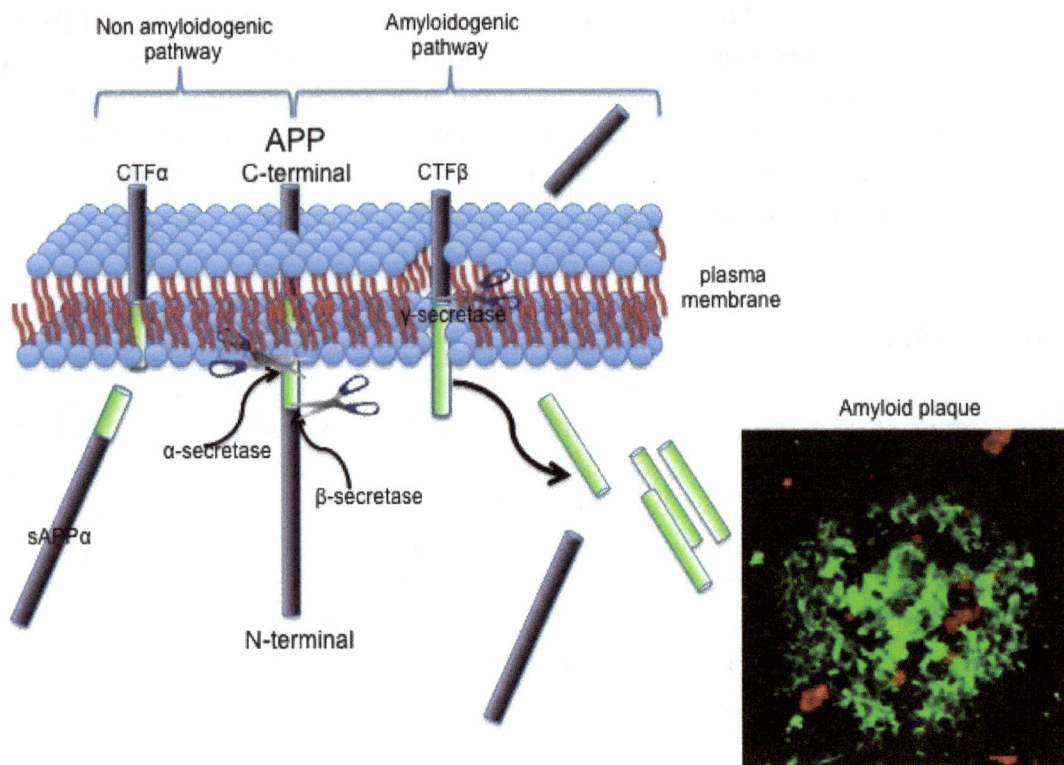

Figure 4. Amyloid precursor protein structure and metabolism. Schematic representation of APP processing by α-, β-, and γ-secretases. APP processing by secretase activities is divided into the non-amyloidogenic pathway on the left and the amyloidogenic pathway on the right. α- and β-secretase activities cleave APP in its extracellular domain to release respectively a soluble fragment sAPPα or sAPPβ in the extracellular space and generate carboxy-terminal fragments CTFα or CTFβ. These CTFs can subsequently be processed by γ-secretase complex to generate AICD and Aβ. The γ-secretase complex is composed of presenilin, nicastrin (NCT), γ-secretase activating protein (GSAP), pen-2, and aph-1.

6. Oxidative stress and Aβ

It is known that Aβ aggregates promote an inflammatory response, mediated mainly by microglia and astrocytes, which activate pathological signaling pathways, which may lead to neurodegeneration. A long-term activation of the innate immune system, is a mechanism capable of triggering an inflammatory cascade that culminates in cytoskeletal alterations (tau aggregation and formation of PHFs) with neurodegenerative consequences of this hypothesis, it has named "neuroimmunomodulation" [31].

One of these pathological signalling pathways that may lead to neurodegeneration, is oxidative stress, defined as the generation of a large amount of reactive oxygen species (ROS), which are highly harmful, leading to the alteration in the structure of proteins, lipids and nucleic acids and cell death [32]. AD described in the oxidative stress caused by free radicals (FRs). Major FRs in human biology are superoxide (O_2 -), the hydroxyl (OH ·), nitric oxide (NO ·), the thiyl (RS ·) and trichloromethyl (CCl_3 ·). There seem to be an accumulation of iron and aluminum in NPs and CSF [33], which could contribute to this oxidative stress [34].

Under physiological conditions, Aβ could regulate the release of NO, neurotransmitters, and hormones, long term potentiation and promotes cell survival. High levels of NO are generated under conditions of inflammation and may contribute to synaptic dysfunction, oxidation of proteins and lipids; culminating in neuronal death [35, 36] (Figure 5).

In AD, it has been shown that the A ˙ -peptide is able to promote the production of NO in microglia and activated astrocytes [37, 38] the release of proinflammatory cytokines such as IL-1β and TNF-α which contribute to the formation of NO and peroxynitrite [38, 39] and cause changes in proteins and lipids, mitochondrial damage, apoptosis and promotes the formation of Aβ, as well as increasing γ-secretase activity [40, 41] (Figure 3, 5). NO synthesis during development of AD could also contribute to the formation of NFTs (Fig 5), favouring the increase of tau phosphorylation [42].

7. Neuroinflammation as a trigger of neuronal death

Inflammation is involved in many pathological mechanisms in AD [43]. Clinicopathological and neuroimaging studies show that microglial activation and inflammation precede neuronal damage [44], and oxidative stress occurs before the histopathologycal lesion of AD appear [45]. But inflammation can be neuroprotective in its early stages [46] and the inability to resolve the activating stimulus can result in a chronic inflammatory response.

Under physiological conditions, glial cells and neurons express cytokines involved in modulating various functions including cellular homeostasis, metabolism, synaptic plasticity, and neural transmission. The Aβ plays a role in synaptic function and pathology [47], inducing degeneration, promoting the release of excitatory neurotransmitters by increasing intracellular calcium and ROS production (Figure 4) [48]. Aβ accumulation in the brain parenchyma and blood vessels promote microglial migration causing chronic and acute inflammatory response and induces production of FRs, proinflammatory cytokines and prostaglandins (PG), which may eventually promote neuronal death [49]. Aβ accumulation could disrupt the normal operation of the neurons, resulting in a significant cell dysfunction, which leads to apoptosis even before the formation of NPs and NFTs.

8. Glial cells key mediators of the inflammatory response in AD

Microglia cells are derived from monocytes during embryogenesis and are responsible for neuronal damage response [49]. Functions related to the immune response participate in a variety of neuroinflammatory processes [50].

The inflammatory response in AD includes morphological changes of microglia cells ranging from a branched cell "inactive" to the amoeboid appearance "active" [51, 52]. Activated microglia expresses several molecules on their surface, such as: Fc receptors required in phagocytosis of opsonized antigens by IgG, scavenger receptors [53], cytokine and chemokine receptors, complement receptors as CD11b, CD11c, CD14, molecules of the major histocompatibility complex (MHC) [54], Toll-like receptors (TLR) family and Aβ receptors as the receptor for advanced glycation endproducts (RAGE). Cell surface microglial receptors are required for interaction with different types of immune cells, molecules involved in inflammatory responses in the brain and Aβ [55-57].

Aβ itself, causes activation of microglia and astrocytes through TLRs 2, 4 and 9 [54], when activated microglial cells produces neurotoxic molecules and strategically are located in the vicinity of the NPs. This proinflammatory cascade generated by microglial activation results in the release of cytotoxic molecules such as interleukins (IL-1 α, IL-1 β, IL-6, IL-10, IL-12, IL-16, IL-23), growth factors (transforming growth factor beta. TGF-β), chemokines, metalloproteinases (MMP-2, MMP-3, MMP-9), eicosanoids (PGD 2, leukotriene C4, cathepsins B and L) and complement factors (C1, C3, C4) also causing astrocytes chemotaxis around NPs [52]. Activated microglia also releases excessive amounts of glutamate and thereby inducing neurodegeneration These molecules can enhance cytotoxic neurodegeneration, increasing sensitivity to FRs [39]. Thus microglia-mediated neurotoxicity depends on ROS and cytokines [58, 59].

9. Astrocytic activation and their significance in the AD

Astrocytes represent the most abundant glial cell type in the CNS. They provide physical and metabolic support for neurons, and they are involved in the formation and maintenance of the BBB (Fig 5A), they produce neurotrophic and neuroprotective factors and are involved in repair processes within the CNS [60]. Attenuate the production of FRs and tumor necrosis factor α (TNF-α) [61], reduces microglial activation by Aβ [62] and alter their phagocytic activity [63]. They also decrease the cytotoxicity of A •, both directly and indirectly through modulation of microglial cells [64].

In early stages of AD, activated astrocytes are located in two areas: in the molecular layer of the cerebral cortex and the amyloid deposits below the pyramidal cell layer. The activated astrocytes can phagocyte and degrade Aβ, suggesting that these cells are very important in the removal of parenchymal Aβ aggregates (Fig 5A and 6A. Arrowheads). As microglia, astrocytes are also activated by TLRs dependent pathways and RAGE receptors, therefore causing local inflammation and eventually favouring neuronal death [49]. Activated astrocytes produce numerous pro-inflammatory molecules as microglia, but unlike microglia, astrocytes produce S100β, which is highly expressed in the proximity of the Aβ deposits. Prolonged activation of astrocytes has a detrimental impact on neuronal survival and S100β could exacerbate this effect [65].

10. Monocytic cells derived from bone marrow function as a compensatory mechanism to remove amyloid deposits

There are 2 types of phagocytic cells within the CNS that are capable of initiating the innate immune response: microglia and peripheral macrophages [66]. These macrophages are recruited into the CNS by cytokines and chemokines, which are released during the microglial and astrocyte activation able to cross the blood brain barrier (BBB) [49]. Cells derived from bone marrow, can cross the BBB into the CNS and differentiate into microglia, which are located surrounding the amyloid deposits [67, 68]. This finding is very important, since if the resident activated microglia is incompetent to eliminate amyloid deposits, macrophages from the periphery could remove them by phagocytosis [69].

The presence of microvasculature in the brain promotes the release of chemokines such as IL-8, MPC-1, MIP-1, MIP-1α and MIP1-β and thereby promoting differentiation of monocytes into macrophages and migration through the BBB [70]. Analysis of the cerebrospinal fluid (CSF) of AD patients showed an increase in the levels of chemokines such as MCP-1 and IL-8 [71, 72]. In vitro models have demonstrated the ability of (CD4 and CD8) lymphocytes to cross the BBB [73] by increasing the level of MIP-1α.

11. Effect of neuroinflammatory environment on BBB integrity

In AD brains, it has been observed a number of inflammatory reactions, surrounding brain microvasculature, together with A • accumulation, which is associated with a dysfunction of the BBB. Morphological the BBB consists mainly of vascular endothelial cells, and other cellular components secondarily supporting the BBB that include pericytes found in the abluminal basal lamina, the perivascular astrocyte that form extensions towards capillaries around the basal lamina of the capillary wall and microglia.

The permeability and integrity of the BBB is regulated by the endothelial intercellular tight junctions (TJ), that consists of three integral membrane proteins: claudin, occludin and adhesion juntion molecules, as well as some accessory cytoplasmic proteins (ZO1, ZO2, ZO3 and cingulin). Cytoplasmic proteins are linked to actin cytoskeleton primary protein essential for the structural and functional maintenance of the endothelium [74]. While adherent junctions are formed by Vascular endothelium cadherin (VE-cadherin) which is a transmembrane glycoprotein catenin that its main function is to anchor the complex of cadherins and thereby the actin cytoskeleton, but also it is involved in the development of cellular signalling pathways (Figure 5) [75].

During neuroinflammation, leukocytes can infiltrate the brain microenvironment generating high levels of inflammatory mediators such as TNF-α and IFN-γ [76]. Increased levels of TNF-α had been reported not only in endothelial and TJ modulating cytoskeletal rearrangement of brain endothelial cells (BEC) [77, 78], but also by causing an increase in the production of caspase-3 leading BEC to apoptosis [79]. However activation of this caspase 3, not always leads to apoptosis [80] and it has been shown that hypoxia can induce activation of caspases 3 and 9, without inducing neuronal apoptosis [81]. The caspase-3 has been involved in the disassembly of ZO-1 and claudin-5 in TJ regardless of fragmentation during cerebral ischemia (Fig. 5. blood Vessel) [82].

A recent study showed that TNF-α alone or in combination with IFN-γ induces hypermeability, causing the leak of paracellular tracers and also induce degradation of ZO-1. Alterations in the function of brain endothelial cells (BEC) could lead to BBB breakdown, due to high concentrations of cytokines that correlates with expression of caspases 3 and 7 through activation of JNK signalling pathway and protein kinase C (PKC) and an increase in the number of apoptotic cells[83]. Treating peripheral microvascular endothelium with high concentrations of TNF-α and IFN-γ results in a loss focal intercellular adhesion mediated by VE-cadherin generating endothelial rupture areas [76] whereas low concentrations of cytokines, also led to effector caspase activation, increased paracellular flux, and redistribution of zonula occludens-1 and VE-cadherin but failed to induce apoptosis. It was also suggested that cytokines have a dose dependent effect on the BEC. The BEC exposed to high levels of cytokines may be susceptible to caspase-mediated apoptosis and the BEC exposed to low concentrations of cytokine does not undergo apoptosis but results in alterations of the BBB [83].

12. Disruption of the blood-brain barrier as a marker of AD and other dementias

BBB dysfunction is a marker of neuroinflammatory diseases [84]. The BEC are the first physical barrier and expresses CNS binding complexes including TJ, and Adherent Junctions (AJ) [85]. In active inflammatory lesions, focal BEC show abnormalities in the distribution of occludin and ZO-1, including the absence or diffuse immunoreactivity at junctions and an increased immunoreactivity in the cytoplasm [86].

Occludin is vulnerable to the attack of matrix metalloproteinase (MMPs) [87]. MMPs can degrade the basal lamina proteins like fibronectin, laminin, and heparan sulfate after ischemic injury, which helps to break the BBB [88, 89]. It was demonstrated in a study the accumulation of occludin in neurons, astrocytes and microglia in AD, frontotemporal dementia (FTD) and vascular dementia (VaD) [90], suggesting a new function of occludin and proteins of the TJ in the pathogenesis of these dementias.

In this same study it was found that claudin 5 is degraded by MMP2 and MMP9 after ischemic damage, and therefore claudin and occludin were found surrounding astrocytes, but not in brain endothelium after an alteration in the BBB [91]. It is likely that the increase in occluding levels found in astrocytes and neurons in VaD, AD and FTD [90], may be a response to autophagy of TJ proteins by these cells after the rupture of the BBB caused by chronic hypoxia, aberrant angiogenesis or both [92].

13. Blood-brain barrier mechanisms of transport and regulation of brainAβ levels

According to the neural theory, Aβ is produced locally in the brain, in contrast to the vascular theory which suggests that the origin of Aβ comes from the circulation, and that the circulation of soluble Aβ (s- Aβ) may contribute to toxicity when it crosses BEC, which compromises the BBB (figure. 3) [93]. It has been proposed that specific receptors of Aβ are present in human brain capillaries and their distribution in the BEC transport could favour the peptide coupling to the BBB [94]. These receptors include RAGE and SR [95]. It is known that both RAGE and SR are receptors with multiple functions including cell endocytosis and transcytosis of macromolecules. RAGE and SR mediate binding of sA ▪ 1-40 at the apical side of human BBB, and RAGE is also involved in sA ▪ 1-40 transcytosis [94].

It has been shown that the interaction between Aβ/RAGE in the luminal membrane of the BBB participates in; 1). The diffusing of Aβ from the circulation to the brain through the BBB parenchyma, 2) Endothelial NF-KB mediated activation resulting in the secretion of pro-inflammatory cytokines (TNF-α and IL-6) and adhesion molecules expression (ICAM-1 and VCAM) and 3), generation of endothelin-1 decreases cerebral blood flow (CBF). The peptide Aβ / RAGE interaction contributes directly to neuronal death producing oxidative damage to neurons expressing RAGE and indirectly through activation of microglia [95]. Inhibition of RAGE/Aβ interaction in affected vasculature inhibits the production of cytokines, oxidative stress and Aβ peptide transport across the BBB [96]. Therefore it is suggested that RAGE could be an excellent therapeutic target in AD. It has been shown that RAGE inhibitors block its interaction to Aβ peptide and stabilizes the BBB functions, reducing neuroinflammation and improving the CBF.

14. Alterations of the neurovascular unit in AD

As previously described Aβ aggregates activate microglia and astrocytes, promoting the secretion of cytotoxic and pro-inflammatory factors culminating in neuronal and BBB dysfunction. Aβ can accumulate in the cerebral blood vessels, causing a morphofunctional alteration of neurovascular function.

Human brain receives 20% of the total cardiac output, if the cerebral blood flow (CBF) is stopped, so do brain functions in seconds and damage to neurons occurs in minutes [97]. The neuron-vessel relationship is critical for normal brain function. It has been estimated that each neuron in the human brain has its own capillary [98].

The length of brain capillaries is reduced in AD. These reductions can decrease vascular transport of substrates and nutrients through the BBB and reduce disposal of neurotoxins [99]. Vascular cells can directly affect the synaptic and neuronal functions through alterations in blood flow, the permeability of the BBB, nutrient supply, removal of toxic molecules, enzymatic functions, secretion of trophic factors and matrix molecules or through abnormal expression of vascular receptors [100]. In response to vascular injury, astrocites and microglia are recruited, which when activated secrete several pro-inflammatory cytokines [101], that in turn, damage and exacerbates neuronal and synaptic dysfunction.

15. Stages of neurovascular dysfunction in AD

In early stages of AD, Aβ peptide removal through the BBB is impair, which could favour the accumulation of neurotoxic Aβ oligomers in the brain. Moreover, Aβ oligomers and focal reduction in capillary blood flow may affect synaptic transmission, causing neuronal damage and initiate the recruitment of microglial cells or blood within the brain [100].

In the early AD symptomatic stage, the BBB start missing Aβ removal properties, and activated endothelium and pro-inflammatory cytokines secreted to the CBF. This increases synaptic dysfunction, accumulation of intracellular tangles and activation of microglia. In late symptomatic AD stages, capillary unit is impair and contribute to the degeneration of the endothelial barrier. At this stage, there is a severe loss of the ability of the BBB to remove Aβ, resulting in amyloid deposits formation in the outer side of the capillary membrane, an increase in the number of NFT and activated microglia and astrocytes. At the final AD stages, the capillary unit is lost due to the amyloid deposits, therefore altering neuronal synapsis (Figure 6) [100].

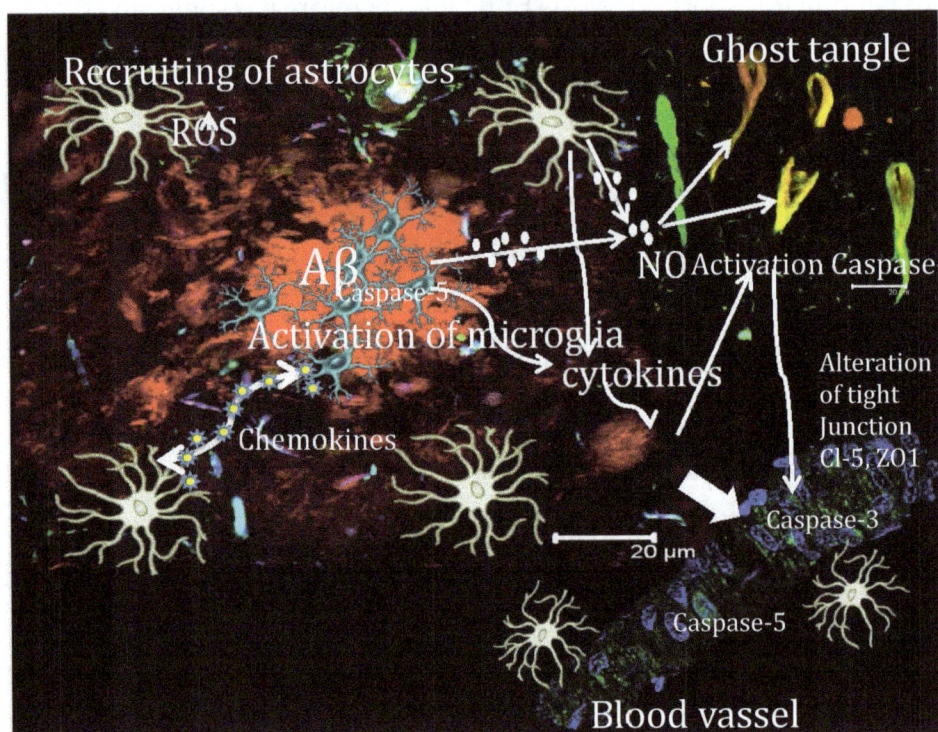

Figure 5. Schematic representation of neuroinflammatory environment and BBB alterations in AD. Aβ aggregates activate microglia and astrocytes, which will secrete pro-inflammatory cytokines and cytotoxic factors that will cause neuronal damage and disruption of the BBB (See more details in text).

16. Brain microvascular dysfunction as early event in AD

It is proposed that the breakdown of the BBB might be directly responsible for the pathogenesis of sporadic AD or at least could participate synergistically with other pathogenic mechanisms in the development of dementia [102]. Altering the BBB might occur as a result of hypoxia and complication of ischemic events, causing myocardial alterations commonly observed in AD. The breakdown of the BBB in AD is supported by the anatomical thickness and functional changes in the cerebral microvasculature [102] Deposits of A • in the cerebral vasculature, leading to thickening of the basement membrane, stenosis of the vessel lumen and fragmentation of the internal elastic lamina, which can lead to stroke, brain haemorrhage or dementia [103, 104].

In AD there are ultrastructural changes [105] in the capillaries and changes in the its distribution and density [106]. It is believed that the accumulation of Aβ is one of the earliest events causing cerebrovascular alterations [107]. It has been detected changes in microvascular permeability and BBB dysfunction in AD brains [108]. BBB regulates the input of plasma derived Aβ and eliminates CNS Aβ through RAGE and the low-density lipoprotein receptor-related protein, (LRP1) respectively [95, 109].

The soluble peptide Aβ (s- Aβ) is normally produced by different cell types [110] and could be released into the circulation of the cerebrospinal fluid (CSF)[9] and brain parenchyma [111]. The Aβ 1-40 peptide represents about 90% of the total cerebrovascular amyloid [112]. High levels of Aβ and the presence of predisposing factors such as apoE4, genetic mutations in PS-1, PS-2 and APP [113], may favor the accumulation of Aβ as fibrillar amyloid in the wall vessel or in the brain parenchyma and could induce cytotoxic effects [95, 114] and contribute to neuronal loss and the development of the AD pathology [113].

Recent studies support the vascular theory to show that the brain distribution of Aβ receptors in the apical side of the BBB might be responsible for the interaction of Aβ circulating with the vascular wall and mediate its transit to the brain [115]. In AD many Aβ deposits are associated with microvessels [116] and with the presence of multiple inflammatory molecules that provide support for monocyte transmigration ability to neighbourhoods of Aβ deposit and in accordance with the clinical- pathological it has been suggested that neuroinflammation plays a role in patients with AD dementia [117]. In a study it was shown that Aβ peptide induced monocyte differentiation into macrophages and hypersecretion of inflammatory cytokines and chemokines [70]. In AD brains, a large number of core amyloid deposits in NPs are intimately associated with endothelial basal lamiña and in many instances the lumen is lost [116]. It has also been found that calcium influx is induced by intracellular Aβ [118, 119], and that elevation of intracellular calcium leads to alteration of the TJ as the induction of MMPs [120].

Chronic transmigration of monocytes may result in subtle damage to the BBB. Disruption of the BBB would allow the passage of large amounts of circulating Aβ linked to other carrier proteins such as albumin [121], α-2 macroglobulin [53] and Aβ components. Albumin levels in CSF of patients with early stages of AD, found to be significantly enhanced due to an increased permeability of the BBB [122]. Elevated levels of other proteins of high molecular weight as haptoglobin, had also been found in this conditions [123].

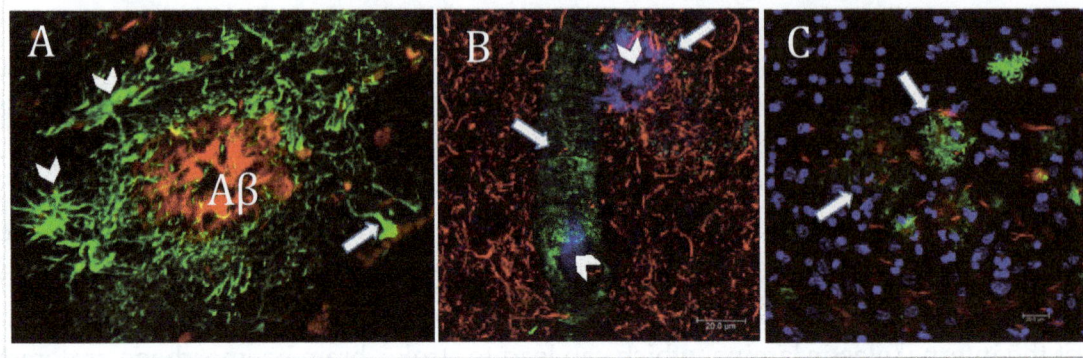

Figure 6. The extracellular deposits of amyloid-β peptide induces cronic inflammation in neuronal cell. A) Double immunostaining. Glial cell immunostaining evidenced by GFAP antibody (arrowheads), which is located in the perifery of the extracellular amyloid deposit evidenced by the thiazine red dye (Aβ). Microglial cell associated with a blood vessel. B) Triple immunostaining, where expression of caspase-5 (green channel) was detected in the cytoplasm of endothelial cells (the blood vessel, arrow). Adjacent to the blood vessel is possible to observed a extracellular Aβ deposit (amyloid plaque) evidenced by antibody BAM10 (arrowheads). In the red channel is the immunoreactivity of an antibody against tau protein. C) Double immunostaining with antibodies raised to Caspase-5 (green channel, arrows), which is strongly associated with amyloid plaques (as evidenced by the thiazine red staining, red channel), counterstained with Topro dye to show cell nuclei (blue channel). confocal microscopy, Leica SP8.

17. Amyloid beta peptide and intracellular caspase 5 in brain endothelial cells

Caspase-5 is expressed in a restricted manner in placenta, lung, liver, spleen, small intestine, colon and peripheral blood lymphocytes (1, 3) and it is located in the cell cytoplasm. It belongs to the family of proteins involved in apoptosis, inflammation, proliferation and differentiation. Caspase-5 operatively was associated with the caspases 1, 4 and 12.

Caspase-5 is regulated by lipopolysaccharide (LPS) and interferon-γ. Suggesting that caspase-5 may perform functions in inflammation and innate immune response. Likewise, it is associated with the complex of proteins that constitute the inflammasome. Caspase-5 also participates in IL-1β processing However the presence of caspase-5 and its role in neurodegenerative diseases is unknown.

In this review we have discuss the inflammatory role that is present in AD brains in response to Aβ accumulation and stress induced by this peptide, triggering a response in microglial and astroglial cells. Which are responsible for this inflammatory damage in AD. This proinflammatory cascade generated by microglial activation resulting from the release of cytotoxic molecules such as interleukins (IL-1 α, IL-1 β, IL-6, IL-10, IL-12, IL-16, IL-23), growth factors (transforming growth factor beta [TGF-β]), chemokines, matrix metalloproteinases (MMP-2, MMP-3, MMP-9), eicosanoids (PGD 2, leukotriene C4, cathepsins B and L) and complement factors (C1, C3, C4) also causing astrocytic chemotaxis around NPs (53). Activated microglia also releases excessive amounts of glutamate excitotoxicity, thereby inducing neurodegeneration. So far caspase-5 has been involved in Aβ induced neuroinflammation in AD brains. In our laboratory we have detect the presence of caspase-5 closely associated with Aβ deposits in blood vessels (Fig. 6 B arrows) and Aβ plaques (Fig. 6 B. arrowhead, Fig. 6. C arrows) in AD brains. NPs showed a high immunoreactivity to caspase-5. The presence of caspase-5 was observed in the area where active microglial cells are and poorly observed in the periphery of the NPs where the astroglial cells are (Fig. 6). This does suggest that microglial cells carry out active inflammatory activity and are responsible for the neurotoxic environment observed in AD.

A large numbers of studies have demonstrated an increase of endothelial cells activity in blood vessels. By double and triple immunostaining and confocal microscopy, we have demonstrated the presence of soluble Aβ and fibrillar Aβ (evidenced by the monoclonal antibody BAM10 and stained with thiazine red (TR), which is used to monitor the fibrillar state of tau and Aβ peptide, with a β pleated sheet conformation.) in endothelial cell soma. It is possible that the accumulation of extracellular Aβ peptide could be trigger by caspase-5 activity, causing an increase in the synthesis of IL, therefore modifying the permeability of cerebral blood vessels by altering tight junctions in AD brains. Consequently the presence and activity of caspase-5 could promote the prolonged and sustained inflammation described in AD brains.

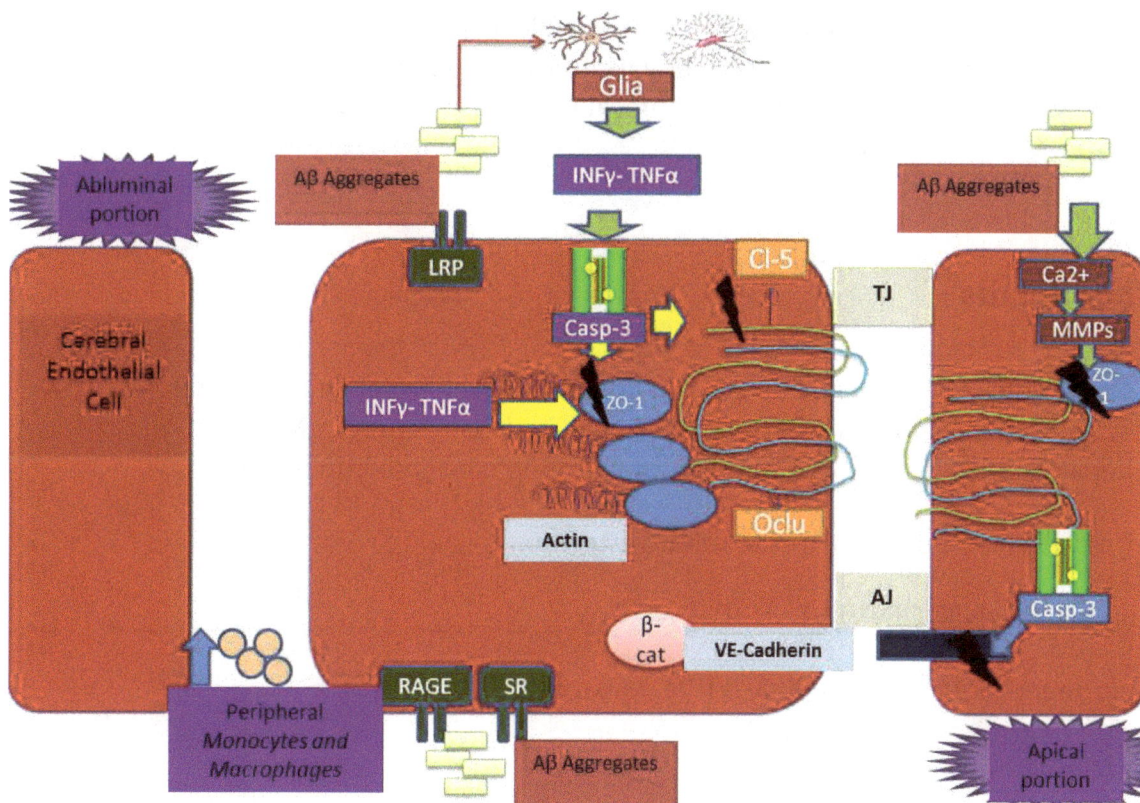

Figure 7. Disruption of the BBB in AD. Aβ aggregates activated glia, pro-inflammatory cytokines secretion, which in turn activate caspase 3, contributing to the disassembly of constitutive adherent junction proteins. The Aβ aggregates also contribute to activation of MMPs. BBB damage, allows monocytes, macrophages and peripheral Aβ aggregated to pass from outside the nervous system to the brain, increasing the neuroinflammatory environment.

18. Conclusions

Amyloid β peptide, which is aggregated extracellularly in the neuritic plaques, generates a constant inflammatory environment and prolonged, activation of microglial and astroglial cells that potentiate neuronal damage and have been involved in the alteration of the BBB, damaging the permeability of blood vessels. Maybe as a consequence of degradation of tight junctions proteins, favouring the loss of these junctions, altering the permeability of blood vessels. Understanding the mechanisms of action of different species of beta amyloid peptide could lead to new therapeutic interventions directed to inhibit Aβ aggregation at the level of oligomers, which are much more toxic than the fibrillary form. It is important to understand the mechanisms of action of caspase-5, in this pathological process of amyloid β peptide, emphasizing the clinical importance of casapasa-5 and its relation to the process of neuroinflammation.

Acknowledgements

The authors wish to express their gratitude to the Mexican families who donate the brain of their loved ones affected with AD and made possible our research. We also want to thank Ms. Maricarmen De Lorenz for her outstanding technical and secretarial support and M en C Ivan J. Galván Mendoza, for hes support in confocal microscopy. This work was supported by the Grant from CONACYT, No. 142293.

Author details

Luis Oskar Soto-Rojas[1,2,3], Fidel de la Cruz-López[2], Miguel Angel Ontiveros Torres[1], Amparo Viramontes-Pintos[1], María del Carmen Cárdenas-Aguayo[4], Marco A. Meraz-Ríos[4], Citlaltepetl Salinas-Lara[3,6], Benjamín Florán-Garduño[5] and José Luna-Muñoz[1*]

*Address all correspondence to: jluna@cinvestav.mx

1 Brain Bank-LaNSE CINVESTAV-IPN, Mexico

2 Departments of Physiology. ENCB IPN, México

3 FES Iztacala. UNAM, México

4 Molecular Biomedicine Department, CINVESTAV-IPN, Mexico

5 Physiology, Biophysics and Neurosciences Department, CINVESTAV-IPN, Mexico

6 INNN MVS, Mexico

References

[1] Ball, M.J., et al., *Neuropathological definition of Alzheimer disease: multivariate analyses in the morphometric distinction between Alzheimer dementia and normal aging.* Alzheimer Dis Assoc Disord, 1988. 2(1): p. 29-37.

[2] Blessed, G., B.E. Tomlinson, and M. Roth, *The association between quantitative measures of dementia and of senile change in the cerebral grey matter of elderly subjects.* Br J Psychiatry, 1968. 114(512): p. 797-811.

[3] Mena, R., et al., *Monitoring pathological assembly of tau and beta-amyloid proteins in Alzheimer's disease.* Acta Neuropathol, 1995. 89(1): p. 50-6.

[4] Cras, P., et al., *Extracellular neurofibrillary tangles reflect neuronal loss and provide further evidence of extensive protein cross-linking in Alzheimer disease.* Acta Neuropathol, 1995. 89(4): p. 291-5.

[5] Gomez-Isla, T., et al., *Neuronal loss correlates with but exceeds neurofibrillary tangles in Alzheimer's disease.* Ann Neurol, 1997. 41(1): p. 17-24.

[6] Gomez-Isla, T., et al., *Profound loss of layer II entorhinal cortex neurons occurs in very mild Alzheimer's disease.* J Neurosci, 1996. 16(14): p. 4491-500.

[7] Bondareff, W., et al., *Evidence of subtypes of Alzheimer's disease and implications for etiology.* Arch Gen Psychiatry, 1993. 50(5): p. 350-6.

[8] Kidd, M., *Paired helical filaments in electron microscopy of Alzheimer's disease.* Nature, 1963. 197: p. 192-3.

[9] Seubert, P., et al., *Isolation and quantification of soluble Alzheimer's beta-peptide from biological fluids.* Nature, 1992. 359(6393): p. 325-7.

[10] Mena, R., et al., *Staging the pathological assembly of truncated tau protein into paired helical filaments in Alzheimer's disease.* Acta Neuropathol, 1996. 91(6): p. 633-41.

[11] Neve, R.L., et al., *A cDNA for a human microtubule associated protein 2 epitope in the Alzheimer neurofibrillary tangle.* Brain Res, 1986. 387(2): p. 193-6.

[12] Goedert, M., et al., *Multiple isoforms of human microtubule-associated protein tau: sequences and localization in neurofibrillary tangles of Alzheimer's disease.* Neuron, 1989. 3(4): p. 519-26.

[13] Goedert, M., et al., *Cloning and sequencing of the cDNA encoding an isoform of microtubule-associated protein tau containing four tandem repeats: differential expression of tau protein mRNAs in human brain.* Embo J, 1989. 8(2): p. 393-9.

[14] Sawa, A., et al., *Molecular diversity at the carboxyl terminus of human and rat tau.* Brain Res Mol Brain Res, 1994. 27(1): p. 111-7.

[15] Andreadis, A., W.M. Brown, and K.S. Kosik, *Structure and novel exons of the human tau gene.* Biochemistry, 1992. 31(43): p. 10626-33.

[16] Andreadis, A., J.A. Broderick, and K.S. Kosik, *Relative exon affinities and suboptimal splice site signals lead to non-equivalence of two cassette exons.* Nucleic Acids Res, 1995. 23(17): p. 3585-93.

[17] Kosik, K.S., et al., *Developmentally regulated expression of specific tau sequences.* Neuron, 1989. 2(4): p. 1389-97.

[18] Goedert, M., et al., *Tau proteins of Alzheimer paired helical filaments: abnormal phosphorylation of all six brain isoforms.* Neuron, 1992. 8(1): p. 159-68.

[19] Grundke-Iqbal, I., et al., *Abnormal phosphorylation of the microtubule-associated protein tau (tau) in Alzheimer cytoskeletal pathology.* Proc Natl Acad Sci U S A, 1986. 83(13): p. 4913-7.

[20] Novak, M., J. Kabat, and C.M. Wischik, *Molecular characterization of the minimal protease resistant tau unit of the Alzheimer's disease paired helical filament.* Embo J, 1993. 12(1): p. 365-70.

[21] Luna-Munoz, J., et al., *Earliest stages of tau conformational changes are related to the appearance of a sequence of specific phospho-dependent tau epitopes in Alzheimer's disease.* J Alzheimers Dis, 2007. 12(4): p. 365-75.

[22] Luna-Munoz, J., et al., *Regional conformational change involving phosphorylation of tau protein at the Thr231, precedes the structural change detected by Alz-50 antibody in Alzheimer's disease.* J Alzheimers Dis, 2005. 8(1): p. 29-41.

[23] Arriagada, P.V., et al., *Neurofibrillary tangles but not senile plaques parallel duration and severity of Alzheimer's disease.* Neurology, 1992. 42(3 Pt 1): p. 631-9.

[24] Saunders, A.M., *Apolipoprotein E and Alzheimer disease: an update on genetic and functional analyses.* J Neuropathol Exp Neurol, 2000. 59(9): p. 751-8.

[25] Haass, C., et al., *Amyloid beta-peptide is produced by cultured cells during normal metabolism.* Nature, 1992. 359(6393): p. 322-5.

[26] Shoji, M., et al., *Production of the Alzheimer amyloid beta protein by normal proteolytic processing.* Science, 1992. 258(5079): p. 126-9.

[27] Lemere, C.A., et al., *Sequence of deposition of heterogeneous amyloid beta-peptides and APO E in Down syndrome: implications for initial events in amyloid plaque formation.* Neurobiol Dis, 1996. 3(1): p. 16-32.

[28] Mattson, M.P., et al., *beta-Amyloid precursor protein metabolites and loss of neuronal Ca2+ homeostasis in Alzheimer's disease.* Trends Neurosci, 1993. 16(10): p. 409-14.

[29] Mattson, M.P., et al., *beta-Amyloid peptides destabilize calcium homeostasis and render human cortical neurons vulnerable to excitotoxicity.* J Neurosci, 1992. 12(2): p. 376-89.

[30] Shea, T.B., S. Prabhakar, and F.J. Ekinci, *Beta-amyloid and ionophore A23187 evoke tau hyperphosphorylation by distinct intracellular pathways: differential involvement of the calpain/protein kinase C system.* J Neurosci Res, 1997. 49(6): p. 759-68.

[31] Fernandez, J.A., et al., *The damage signals hypothesis of Alzheimer's disease pathogenesis.* J Alzheimers Dis, 2008. 14(3): p. 329-33.

[32] Lavados, M., et al., *Mild cognitive impairment and Alzheimer patients display different levels of redox-active CSF iron.* J Alzheimers Dis, 2008. 13(2): p. 225-32.

[33] Jellinger, K., et al., *Brain iron and ferritin in Parkinson's and Alzheimer's diseases.* J Neural Transm Park Dis Dement Sect, 1990. 2(4): p. 327-40.

[34] Pappolla, M.A., et al., *Immunohistochemical evidence of oxidative [corrected] stress in Alzheimer's disease.* Am J Pathol, 1992. 140(3): p. 621-8.

[35] Liu, B., et al., *Role of nitric oxide in inflammation-mediated neurodegeneration.* Ann N Y Acad Sci, 2002. 962: p. 318-31.

[36] Calabrese, V., et al., *Nitric oxide in the central nervous system: neuroprotection versus neurotoxicity.* Nat Rev Neurosci, 2007. 8(10): p. 766-75.

[37] Goodwin, J.L., M.E. Kehrli, Jr., and E. Uemura, *Integrin Mac-1 and beta-amyloid in microglial release of nitric oxide.* Brain Res, 1997. 768(1-2): p. 279-86.

[38] Rossi, F. and E. Bianchini, *Synergistic induction of nitric oxide by beta-amyloid and cytokines in astrocytes.* Biochem Biophys Res Commun, 1996. 225(2): p. 474-8.

[39] Combs, C.K., et al., *beta-Amyloid stimulation of microglia and monocytes results in TNFalpha-dependent expression of inducible nitric oxide synthase and neuronal apoptosis.* J Neurosci, 2001. 21(4): p. 1179-88.

[40] Keil, U., et al., *Amyloid beta-induced changes in nitric oxide production and mitochondrial activity lead to apoptosis.* J Biol Chem, 2004. 279(48): p. 50310-20.

[41] Guix, F.X., et al., *Modification of gamma-secretase by nitrosative stress links neuronal ageing to sporadic Alzheimer's disease.* EMBO Mol Med, 2012. 4(7): p. 660-73.

[42] Saez, T.E., et al., *Astrocytic nitric oxide triggers tau hyperphosphorylation in hippocampal neurons.* In Vivo, 2004. 18(3): p. 275-80.

[43] McGeer, P.L. and E.G. McGeer, *Inflammation, autotoxicity and Alzheimer disease.* Neurobiol Aging, 2001. 22(6): p. 799-809.

[44] Eikelenboom, P. and W.A. van Gool, *Neuroinflammatory perspectives on the two faces of Alzheimer's disease.* J Neural Transm, 2004. 111(3): p. 281-94.

[45] Zhu, X., et al., *Alzheimer's disease: the two-hit hypothesis.* Lancet Neurol, 2004. 3(4): p. 219-26.

[46] Wyss-Coray, T., et al., *Prominent neurodegeneration and increased plaque formation in complement-inhibited Alzheimer's mice.* Proc Natl Acad Sci U S A, 2002. 99(16): p. 10837-42.

[47] Kamenetz, F., et al., *APP processing and synaptic function.* Neuron, 2003. 37(6): p. 925-37.

[48] Gylys, K.H., et al., *Synaptic changes in Alzheimer's disease: increased amyloid-beta and gliosis in surviving terminals is accompanied by decreased PSD-95 fluorescence.* Am J Pathol, 2004. 165(5): p. 1809-17.

[49] Meraz-Rios, M.A., et al., *Inflammatory process in Alzheimer's Disease.* Front Integr Neurosci, 2013. 7: p. 59.

[50] Lund, S., et al., *The dynamics of the LPS triggered inflammatory response of murine microglia under different culture and in vivo conditions.* J Neuroimmunol, 2006. 180(1-2): p. 71-87.

[51] Suh, Y.H. and F. Checler, *Amyloid precursor protein, presenilins, and alpha-synuclein: molecular pathogenesis and pharmacological applications in Alzheimer's disease.* Pharmacol Rev, 2002. 54(3): p. 469-525.

[52] Glass, C.K., et al., *Mechanisms underlying inflammation in neurodegeneration.* Cell, 2010. 140(6): p. 918-34.

[53] Hughes, S.R., et al., *Alpha2-macroglobulin associates with beta-amyloid peptide and prevents fibril formation.* Proc Natl Acad Sci U S A, 1998. 95(6): p. 3275-80.

[54] Suzumura, A., *[Neurotoxicity by microglia: the mechanisms and potential therapeutic strategy].* Fukuoka Igaku Zasshi, 2009. 100(7): p. 243-7.

[55] El Khoury, J., et al., *Scavenger receptor-mediated adhesion of microglia to beta-amyloid fibrils.* Nature, 1996. 382(6593): p. 716-9.

[56] Lue, L.F., et al., *Involvement of microglial receptor for advanced glycation endproducts (RAGE) in Alzheimer's disease: identification of a cellular activation mechanism.* Exp Neurol, 2001. 171(1): p. 29-45.

[57] McGeer, P.L., et al., *Microglia in degenerative neurological disease.* Glia, 1993. 7(1): p. 84-92.

[58] Benzing, W.C., et al., *Evidence for glial-mediated inflammation in aged APP(SW) transgenic mice.* Neurobiol Aging, 1999. 20(6): p. 581-9.

[59] Mehlhorn, G., M. Hollborn, and R. Schliebs, *Induction of cytokines in glial cells surrounding cortical beta-amyloid plaques in transgenic Tg2576 mice with Alzheimer pathology.* Int J Dev Neurosci, 2000. 18(4-5): p. 423-31.

[60] Minagar, A., et al., *The role of macrophage/microglia and astrocytes in the pathogenesis of three neurologic disorders: HIV-associated dementia, Alzheimer disease, and multiple sclerosis.* J Neurol Sci, 2002. 202(1-2): p. 13-23.

[61] Smits, H.A., et al., *Activation of human macrophages by amyloid-beta is attenuated by astrocytes.* J Immunol, 2001. 166(11): p. 6869-76.

[62] von Bernhardi, R. and G. Ramirez, *Microglia-astrocyte interaction in Alzheimer's disease: friends or foes for the nervous system?* Biol Res, 2001. 34(2): p. 123-8.

[63] DeWitt, D.A., et al., *Astrocytes regulate microglial phagocytosis of senile plaque cores of Alzheimer's disease.* Exp Neurol, 1998. 149(2): p. 329-40.

[64] Ramirez, G., et al., *Protection of rat primary hippocampal cultures from A beta cytotoxicity by pro-inflammatory molecules is mediated by astrocytes.* Neurobiol Dis, 2005. 19(1-2): p. 243-54.

[65] Mori, T., et al., *Overexpression of human S100B exacerbates cerebral amyloidosis and gliosis in the Tg2576 mouse model of Alzheimer's disease.* Glia, 2010. 58(3): p. 300-14.

[66] Rezai-Zadeh, K., D. Gate, and T. Town, *CNS infiltration of peripheral immune cells: D-Day for neurodegenerative disease?* J Neuroimmune Pharmacol, 2009. 4(4): p. 462-75.

[67] Malm, T.M., et al., *Bone-marrow-derived cells contribute to the recruitment of microglial cells in response to beta-amyloid deposition in APP/PS1 double transgenic Alzheimer mice.* Neurobiol Dis, 2005. 18(1): p. 134-42.

[68] Simard, A.R., et al., *Bone marrow-derived microglia play a critical role in restricting senile plaque formation in Alzheimer's disease.* Neuron, 2006. 49(4): p. 489-502.

[69] Gate, D., et al., *Macrophages in Alzheimer's disease: the blood-borne identity.* J Neural Transm, 2010. 117(8): p. 961-70.

[70] Fiala, M., et al., *Amyloid-beta induces chemokine secretion and monocyte migration across a human blood--brain barrier model.* Mol Med, 1998. 4(7): p. 480-9.

[71] Galimberti, D., et al., *Chemokines in serum and cerebrospinal fluid of Alzheimer's disease patients.* Ann Neurol, 2003. 53(4): p. 547-8.

[72] Correa, J.D., et al., *Chemokines in CSF of Alzheimer's disease patients.* Arq Neuropsiquiatr, 2011. 69(3): p. 455-9.

[73] Man, S.M., et al., *Peripheral T cells overexpress MIP-1alpha to enhance its transendothelial migration in Alzheimer's disease.* Neurobiol Aging, 2007. 28(4): p. 485-96.

[74] Tsukita, S. and M. Furuse, *Occludin and claudins in tight-junction strands: leading or supporting players?* Trends Cell Biol, 1999. 9(7): p. 268-73.

[75] Stamatovic, S.M., R.F. Keep, and A.V. Andjelkovic, *Brain endothelial cell-cell junctions: how to "open" the blood brain barrier.* Curr Neuropharmacol, 2008. 6(3): p. 179-92.

[76] Wong, R.K., A.L. Baldwin, and R.L. Heimark, *Cadherin-5 redistribution at sites of TNF-alpha and IFN-gamma-induced permeability in mesenteric venules.* Am J Physiol, 1999. 276(2 Pt 2): p. H736-48.

[77] Forster, C., et al., *Differential effects of hydrocortisone and TNFalpha on tight junction proteins in an in vitro model of the human blood-brain barrier.* J Physiol, 2008. 586(7): p. 1937-49.

[78] de Vries, H.E., et al., *The influence of cytokines on the integrity of the blood-brain barrier in vitro.* J Neuroimmunol, 1996. 64(1): p. 37-43.

[79] Kimura, H., et al., *Cytotoxicity of cytokines in cerebral microvascular endothelial cell.* Brain Res, 2003. 990(1-2): p. 148-56.

[80] Kroemer, G. and S.J. Martin, *Caspase-independent cell death.* Nat Med, 2005. 11(7): p. 725-30.

[81] Garnier, P., et al., *Hypoxia induces caspase-9 and caspase-3 activation without neuronal death in gerbil brains.* Eur J Neurosci, 2004. 20(4): p. 937-46.

[82] Zehendner, C.M., et al., *Caspase-3 contributes to ZO-1 and Cl-5 tight-junction disruption in rapid anoxic neurovascular unit damage.* PLoS One, 2011. 6(2): p. e16760.

[83] Lopez-Ramirez, M.A., et al., *Role of caspases in cytokine-induced barrier breakdown in human brain endothelial cells.* J Immunol, 2012. 189(6): p. 3130-9.

[84] McQuaid, S., et al., *The effects of blood-brain barrier disruption on glial cell function in multiple sclerosis.* Biochem Soc Trans, 2009. 37(Pt 1): p. 329-31.

[85] Ballabh, P., A. Braun, and M. Nedergaard, *The blood-brain barrier: an overview: structure, regulation, and clinical implications.* Neurobiol Dis, 2004. 16(1): p. 1-13.

[86] Plumb, J., et al., *Abnormal endothelial tight junctions in active lesions and normal-appearing white matter in multiple sclerosis.* Brain Pathol, 2002. 12(2): p. 154-69.

[87] Rosenberg, G.A. and Y. Yang, *Vasogenic edema due to tight junction disruption by matrix metalloproteinases in cerebral ischemia.* Neurosurg Focus, 2007. 22(5): p. E4.

[88] Cheng, T., et al., *Activated protein C inhibits tissue plasminogen activator-induced brain hemorrhage.* Nat Med, 2006. 12(11): p. 1278-85.

[89] Zlokovic, B.V., *Remodeling after stroke.* Nat Med, 2006. 12(4): p. 390-1.

[90] Romanitan, M.O., et al., *Occludin is overexpressed in Alzheimer's disease and vascular dementia.* J Cell Mol Med, 2007. 11(3): p. 569-79.

[91] Yang, Y., et al., *Matrix metalloproteinase-mediated disruption of tight junction proteins in cerebral vessels is reversed by synthetic matrix metalloproteinase inhibitor in focal ischemia in rat.* J Cereb Blood Flow Metab, 2007. 27(4): p. 697-709.

[92] Wu, Z., et al., *Role of the MEOX2 homeobox gene in neurovascular dysfunction in Alzheimer disease.* Nat Med, 2005. 11(9): p. 959-65.

[93] Zlokovic, B., *Can blood-brain barrier play a role in the development of cerebral amyloidosis and Alzheimer's disease pathology.* Neurobiol Dis, 1997. 4(1): p. 23-6.

[94] Mackic, J.B., et al., *Human blood-brain barrier receptors for Alzheimer's amyloid-beta 1- 40. Asymmetrical binding, endocytosis, and transcytosis at the apical side of brain microvascular endothelial cell monolayer.* J Clin Invest, 1998. 102(4): p. 734-43.

[95] Yan, S.D., et al., *RAGE and amyloid-beta peptide neurotoxicity in Alzheimer's disease.* Nature, 1996. 382(6593): p. 685-91.

[96] Deane, R., et al., *RAGE mediates amyloid-beta peptide transport across the blood-brain barrier and accumulation in brain.* Nat Med, 2003. 9(7): p. 907-13.

[97] Girouard, H. and C. Iadecola, *Neurovascular coupling in the normal brain and in hypertension, stroke, and Alzheimer disease.* J Appl Physiol (1985), 2006. 100(1): p. 328-35.

[98] Zlokovic, B.V., *Neurovascular mechanisms of Alzheimer's neurodegeneration.* Trends Neurosci, 2005. 28(4): p. 202-8.

[99] Bailey, T.L., et al., *The nature and effects of cortical microvascular pathology in aging and Alzheimer's disease.* Neurol Res, 2004. 26(5): p. 573-8.

[100] Zlokovic, B.V., *The blood-brain barrier in health and chronic neurodegenerative disorders.* Neuron, 2008. 57(2): p. 178-201.

[101] Man, S., E.E. Ubogu, and R.M. Ransohoff, *Inflammatory cell migration into the central nervous system: a few new twists on an old tale.* Brain Pathol, 2007. 17(2): p. 243-50.

[102] Buee, L., P.R. Hof, and A. Delacourte, *Brain microvascular changes in Alzheimer's disease and other dementias.* Ann N Y Acad Sci, 1997. 826: p. 7-24.

[103] Weller, R.O. and J.A. Nicoll, *Cerebral amyloid angiopathy: both viper and maggot in the brain.* Ann Neurol, 2005. 58(3): p. 348-50.

[104] Rensink, A.A., et al., *Pathogenesis of cerebral amyloid angiopathy.* Brain Res Brain Res Rev, 2003. 43(2): p. 207-23.

[105] Vinters, H.V., et al., *Microvasculature in brain biopsy specimens from patients with Alzheimer's disease: an immunohistochemical and ultrastructural study.* Ultrastruct Pathol, 1994. 18(3): p. 333-48.

[106] Kalaria, R.N. and P. Hedera, *Differential degeneration of the cerebral microvasculature in Alzheimer's disease.* Neuroreport, 1995. 6(3): p. 477-80.

[107] Selkoe, D.J., *Alzheimer's disease: genes, proteins, and therapy.* Physiol Rev, 2001. 81(2): p. 741-66.

[108]   Claudio, L., *Ultrastructural features of the blood-brain barrier in biopsy tissue from Alzheimer's disease patients.* Acta Neuropathol, 1996. 91(1): p. 6-14.

[109]   Shibata, M., et al., *Clearance of Alzheimer's amyloid-ss(1-40) peptide from brain by LDL receptor-related protein-1 at the blood-brain barrier.* J Clin Invest, 2000. 106(12): p. 1489-99.

[110]   Citron, M., et al., *Evidence that the 42- and 40-amino acid forms of amyloid beta protein are generated from the beta-amyloid precursor protein by different protease activities.* Proc Natl Acad Sci U S A, 1996. 93(23): p. 13170-5.

[111]   Tabaton, M., et al., *Soluble amyloid beta-protein is a marker of Alzheimer amyloid in brain but not in cerebrospinal fluid.* Biochem Biophys Res Commun, 1994. 200(3): p. 1598-603.

[112]   Masters, C.L., et al., *Amyloid plaque core protein in Alzheimer disease and Down syndrome.* Proc Natl Acad Sci U S A, 1985. 82(12): p. 4245-9.

[113]   Wisniewski, T., J. Ghiso, and B. Frangione, *Biology of A beta amyloid in Alzheimer's disease.* Neurobiol Dis, 1997. 4(5): p. 313-28.

[114]   Mattson, M.P. and R.E. Rydel, *Alzheimer's disease. Amyloid ox-tox transducers.* Nature, 1996. 382(6593): p. 674-5.

[115]   Thomas, T., et al., *beta-Amyloid-mediated vasoactivity and vascular endothelial damage.* Nature, 1996. 380(6570): p. 168-71.

[116]   Roher, A.E., et al., *beta-Amyloid-(1-42) is a major component of cerebrovascular amyloid deposits: implications for the pathology of Alzheimer disease.* Proc Natl Acad Sci U S A, 1993. 90(22): p. 10836-40.

[117]   Mirra, S.S., M.N. Hart, and R.D. Terry, *Making the diagnosis of Alzheimer's disease. A primer for practicing pathologists.* Arch Pathol Lab Med, 1993. 117(2): p. 132-44.

[118]   Griffin, W.S., et al., *Interleukin-1 expression in different plaque types in Alzheimer's disease: significance in plaque evolution.* J Neuropathol Exp Neurol, 1995. 54(2): p. 276-81.

[119]   Hull, M., et al., *Occurrence of interleukin-6 in cortical plaques of Alzheimer's disease patients may precede transformation of diffuse into neuritic plaques.* Ann N Y Acad Sci, 1996. 777: p. 205-12.

[120]   Quintanilla, R.A., et al., *Interleukin-6 induces Alzheimer-type phosphorylation of tau protein by deregulating the cdk5/p35 pathway.* Exp Cell Res, 2004. 295(1): p. 245-57.

[121]   Biere, A.L., et al., *Amyloid beta-peptide is transported on lipoproteins and albumin in human plasma.* J Biol Chem, 1996. 271(51): p. 32916-22.

[122]   Mecocci, P., et al., *Blood-brain-barrier in a geriatric population: barrier function in degenerative and vascular dementias.* Acta Neurol Scand, 1991. 84(3): p. 210-3.

[123]   Mattila, K.M., et al., Altered blood-brain-barrier function in Alzheimer's disease? Acta Neurol Scand, 1994. 89(3): p. 192-8.

6

New Frontiers in Alzheimer's Disease Diagnosis

Franc Llorens, Sabine Nuhn, Christoph Peter,
Inga Zerr and Katharina Stoeck

Additional information is available at the end of the chapter

1. Introduction

Alzheimer´s disease (AD) is the most prevalent form of dementia accounting for 60-70% of all cases worldwide. As the world's population ages the incidence of AD is expected to increase rapidly turning into a global epidemic disease with incalculable sociological and economic consequences. In 2006, the prevalence of AD worldwide was calculated in 26.6 million and it is estimated that by 2050 current prevalence will be triplicated or quadruplicated, affecting 1 out of 85 persons worldwide [1, 2]. An accurate diagnosis and a timely detection are critical for improving the physical, clinical, emotional and financial impacts of the disease. However, this aim is far to be achieved and several studies indicate that less than 35 percentage of people living with AD or related dementias are correctly diagnosed [3, 4]. As a consequence, between 18% and 67% of the dementia patients are treated with a potentially inappropriate medication [5].

In this dramatic scenario, new technical, methodological and notional approaches are explored in order to overcome the inherent limitations in AD clinical diagnosis. Indeed, the identification of reliable diagnostic tools in AD remains impeded by the clinical, neuropathological and molecular overlap existing between AD and other types of dementia such as Mild Cognitive Impairment (MCI), or mixed forms of dementia, such as Vascular Dementia (VaD), Fronto-temporal Lobar Degeneration (FTLD) or Lewy Body Dementia (LBD), and by the high AD heterogeneity according to disease onset, progression and duration [6-8].

Since the complexity of this scenario impairs the use of current diagnostic tools for a correct data interpretation, in the recent years, new strategies such as the integrated and combined use of neuropsychological profiles, imaging and biological fluids biomarkers have been developed, improving current diagnosis classification [9-11] and predicting the conversion from MCI to AD [12, 13].

Despite recent solid advances in the topic, up to date, no single diagnostic tool or combination of diagnostic tools can unequivocally confirm AD diagnosis. Indeed absolute confirmation and definite AD diagnostic still requires histopathologic analysis on the post-mortem brain certifying the presence of the pathologic disease hallmarks such as β-amyloid plaques and neurofibrillary tangles.

Since AD is a progressive disease and no treatment is available to recover neuronal integrity, the inaccuracy of AD early diagnosis and prognosis makes early therapeutic intervention difficult and impedes the prevention of neurodegeneration and cognitive dysfunction.

Identification of disease specific clinical, imaging and biochemical-based tools at early stages will help to greater extent to an early treatment which may restrain the disease progression. Additionally, a thorough understanding of the role of biomarkers in AD disease and their modulated levels in AD patients will facilitate the comprehension of their role in AD etiopathology and would help to establish a link between diagnostic and therapeutic fields. Therefore, the ultimate goal is to develop early and reliable diagnosis methods to establish an appropriate and prompt treatment. Indeed this aspect is imperative to maximize the efficiency of potential therapies and decrease symptomatology before pathological changes spread throughout the brain and massive death of neurons has already occurred. Finally, it should also be taken into consideration that the development of successful epidemiological risk assessment and diagnosis programs, including a routinely monitoring of disease progression, will need to be established through the development of new methodologies and protocols at low cost and with non-invasive approaches.

The present chapter summarizes the most recent findings in the field of AD, including neuropsychological profiles and brain and biological fluids biomarkers, which are currently paving the way for new focused approaches in AD diagnosis and prognosis.

2. Diagnostic criteria/Clinical and research criteria

According to the International Classification of Diseases (ICD-10) and the Diagnostic and Statistical Manual of Mental Disorders of the American Psychiatric Association (DSM IV) dementia is defined as a a worsening of cognitive function from a preexisting individual level. The major symptom is decline in memory and should be followed by at least one dysfunction in another major cognitive core skill, severe enough to impair a person's ability to perform everyday activities. The cognitive impairments should be irreversible and not be attributable to e.g. a delirium or another psychiatric disorder and must be present for at least 6 month.

Moreover, the German Society of Psychiatry, Psychotherapy and Neurology (DGPPN) as well as the German Neurological Society (DGN) refer to a subtle change in personality and behavior in the process of dementia [14]. The criteria of the American National Institute of Neurological and Communicative Disorders and Stroke/Alzheimer's disease and Related Disorders Association (NINCDS/ADRDA) are more often referred to in the literature, which differentiate the degree of diagnostic accuracy in "possible" or "probable dementia" [15, 16].

Based on the latter, commonly accepted dementia criteria, a "probable Alzheimer's dementia" (AD dementia) is diagnosed by signs of dementia on clinical examination and neuropsychological tests whereby the memory impairment should be followed by another deficit in an additional cognitive skill. In alternative there is impairment in two cognitive skills with a recognized progression and without evidence of a reduced consciousness.

The age at onset should range between 40 and 90 years and other reasons for the cognitive decline, e.g. treatable causes, should have been carefully ruled out in the diagnostic work up.

The clinical criteria of a "possible Alzheimer's dementia" comprise a dementia syndrome of untypical clinical presentation or duration in absence of other recognizable factors causative of dementia, or if there is a progressive cognitive deficit without a recognized underlying cause.

Exclusion criteria are referred to as sudden onset, focal neurological signs (hemiparesis, hemianopsia) at onset as well as early appearance of gait disorders or epileptic fits.

This categorization is kept according to different revisions of the NINCDS/ADRDA-criteria [16, 17]. Additionally, next to deficits in episodic memory, detection of specific biomarkers in the cerebrospinal fluid (CSF) and imaging (Magnetic Resonance Imaging (MRI) and/or Emission Computed Tomography (PET) is suggested which can increase sensitivity of AD diagnosis.

Further supporting results are, e.g., a progressive worsening of specific cognitive function, disabling in all-day activities, and occurrence of behavioral changes, a positive family history of AD (especially if neuropathologically confirmed), a normal CSF result (basic analysis) and unspecific electroencephalogram (EEG) changes.

A diagnosis of AD is compatible with plateaus during disease course, side symptoms as depression, aggressive behavior, paranoia etc., neurological symptoms in progressed disease state (myoclonus, gait problems, epileptic fits) and a normal Computerized Tomography (CT)-scan [14].

While both terminologies: "probable AD", "possible AD" are proposed for the clinical setting, a third category of "probable and possible AD" was suggested for research purposes. Recent research criteria for clinical AD diagnosis include next to mnestic deficits an occurrence of deficits in non-mnestic function, e.g., language, visual-spatial orientation, executive function. Furthermore, an early diagnosis of AD is proposed already during prodromal stages of dementia, which refer to the clinical picture of a mild cognitive impairment (MCI) [18].

A MCI is a recognized risk factor for AD. Yet, there are presently no commonly agreed criteria [14]. According to international consensus criteria, MCI is considered a condition between normal and demented, a worsening of cognitive function (on self-observation or observation by others) that can be demonstrated on neuropsychological tests, a worsening of cognitive function during an observational time period during disease as well as conserved or only minimally impaired dysfunction in complex all-day activities [19]. The difference between MCI and dementia is based mostly on well-functioning in all-day activities. Standard measurements for cognitive function comprise 1-1.5 standard deviation below the age- and education-matched age group and a mini-mental status test of 24 or above points [18, 20].

The prevalence and conversion rates are variable according to the distinct examination setting. In the clinical setting the annual conversion rate from MCI to AD has been calculated at around 10 percent [14, 21].

At present 4 different MCI subtypes are characterized: amnestic single domain, amnestic multiple domains, non-amnestic single domain and non-amnestic multiple domains [20], whereas the probability to develop AD is highest in MCI with memory deficits [14, 21].

3. Neuropsychological profiles

3.1. The neuropsychological profile of AD

AD is generally characterized by a slowly progressive preclinical (pre-symptomatical) state over several years, an approximately 1-2 years lasting pre-dementia phase until development of dementia, which can be categorized into 3 states (mild, medium, severe) [22, 23].

The progressive cognitive deficits hereby parallel neuropathological changes in the brain, whereby cognitive deficits vary individually. The degree of disease severeness refers to cognition and life skills, whereby transition of states can merge. A mild dementia is considered when complex tasks cannot be performed anymore, but an independent life organisation is still possible. A medium-state dementia is referred to if an independent life organisation is impaired but possible with help and observation of family and care-givers. In severe dementia constant guidance and help is required, an independent life organisation is not possible anymore.

At early stages of AD deficits are predominantly characterized by impairment of declarative memory, visual-spatial orientation and lexical-semantic language. Emotionally, in social contacts as well as in personality, patients with AD appear normal for a long period of time ("facade"). They tend to trivialize their deficits. When they recognize cognitive dysfunction, AD patients often describe themselves to be more forgetful without further specification.

Memory impairment (representative brain areas: hippocampus, gyrus parahippocampalis and adjusted temporomedial areas) affects the ability to encode and recapitulate novel memory contents for a longer period of time, whereas the short time memory and the working memory are mostly unaffected in early stages. The procedural memory often keeps unaffected. In the clinical setting progressive memory deficits often appear in forgetfulness of novel information, in repetitive phrases, difficulties in maintaining complex tasks (strands), e.g. forgetting where the keys/money have been stored, which can lead to paranoid reactions. Neuropsychological characterisations are a slow learning curve, rapid forgetfulness, recency-effects due to deficits in encoding, impaired and prolonged memorising, intrusions and a reduced discrimination-ability, non-profit of context cues as well as deficits in orientation in time [22].

In further disease progression according to a time-associated gradient (first in- last out) also long term memories (semantic and biographical memory) are impaired, with affection of identity and personality in medium and severe AD stages [23].

Deficits of the *visual-spatial orientation* (representative brain areas: parietal lobes) are often associates with important all-day activities: writing, calculating, reading the clock, getting dressed or basic orientation in space. This can overlap with memory deficits and deficits in planning skills. Firstly affected are untrained complex skills, e.g., drawing, clock drawing (mispositioning of the minute hand, confusion of hour/minute hand), reading street maps, orientation in unknown buildings, filling in documents. Drawings can show simplifications, repetitions, altered angles, "closing-in" and loss of perspective. Well established and trained skills, e.g., reading, signing a paper, getting dressed, are mainly affected in medium disease stage. A sensitive parameter that can be valuable in early AD diagnosis but also as a parameter of disease progression is clock reading as a trained skill [24, 25].

Deficits in visual-spatial orientation with massive impairment in complex visual awareness are the main characteristic and leading symptom of the *posterior cortical atrophy* (affected brain region: atrophy of the parietal and occipital lobe). The posterior cortical atrophy is a recognised variant of AD with early onset, early visual agnosia and prosopagnosia, whereas memory is less impaired in the beginning [23]. Depending on the affected projection system (occipital-parietal or occipital-temporal) problems of analysing visual-spatial information: e.g., space, depth, movement, position and orientation (dorsal visual route/"where-system") or problems in analysing of shapes/structures, colours, objects, faces and complex space-topographical scenes (ventral visual route/"what system") can occur. Both systems are tightly connected [26, 27].

Affection of *language* (affected brain region: Wernicke area) is characterized by initial difficulties in finding the right words, which is compensated by strategies of avoidance and paraphrases as well as by difficulties in naming of less frequently used objects. The patients tend to make semantic-superior and semantic-associative mistakes (dog=animal, pyramid=Egypt or also volcano=vesuvius). Syntax, articulation and prosody are unaffected.

Material that they read is less often understood, the understanding of complex facts or contents in the figurative sense (collocations) is declining. Verbal fluency is reduced, whereas the semantic is more affected than the phonematic [28]. During disease, language becomes progressively poor of content, stays however relatively fluent with difficulties in word finding as well as with imprecise, diffuse and less informative comments, drifting from topic, talking cross purposes and setting phrases. This results in abrupt sentences, mistakes of syntax, phonematic paraphrases and in problems of speech comprehension for simple comments. In the final stages a total loss of speech occurs [23].

Next to the 3 main symptoms, disturbances in *executive function* (affected brain region: prefrontal cortex) appear. Executive functions comprise: problem solving thinking, monitoring, planning and conducting of complex tasks, working memory, cognitive fluidity and flexibility. Besides a reduced word fluidity and flexibility also abilities in planning can be impaired early. Especially the so-called set-shifting abilities, that require a permanent shift in alertness, are affected at early stages [29].

Attention is tightly associated with executive function. This is especially required in complex tasks. Deficits in attention initially present very discretely, e.g. in dual task-questions (prefrontal cortex, anterior cingulum).

During disease progression, also alertness is impaired which presence of a more rapid exhaustion.

During medium stages all components of attention are majorly affected [22]. Last but not least, apraxia (affected brain region: parietal lobe) and agnosia (affected brain region: occipital lobe and both basal temporal neocortex) can occur already during early and middle stages of dementia. Simple movements are not possible any longer, inaccurate moves cannot be corrected, this can present as, e.g., body-part-as object-mistakes (ideomotoric apraxia), impairment of planning and conducting of sequential tasks (ideatoric apraxia), recognition of line drawing is inhibited.

Cognitive-related *impairment of all-day activities* affects complex instrumental skills in early stages of dementia, e.g. using new instruments, filling in written documents, later on using familiar devices and basal all-day abilities deteriorate progressively.

Psychiatric side symptoms such as anxiety, agitation, excitability, aggressive behaviour or paranoia are not frequently present in early stages, but appear more often in middle and late stages of disease. There is a higher vulnerability for states of disorientation already in the preclinical stage, e.g. after hospital admissions, drug intolerance, malnutrition. Also depressive mood changes as well as reduction of daily activities are considered early signs [23].

Depression is the most frequent psychiatric side symptom and accounts for about 30% of the patients, especially during early disease stage and here from the degree of presentation rather mild. However, depression is considered a main psychiatric disease in the elderly. In general, depressed patients can articulate their symptoms more precisely; they can manage their all-day activities in a better way and demonstrate during neuropsychological testing self-doubts and complain about deficits in concentration. The mood is continuously suppressed and a lack of motivation is more exhibited.

The onset of cognitive deterioration is more distinct in patients with depression, whereas in patients with AD this occurs more gradually. The deficits can affect the whole spectrum of cognition, whereby executive dysfunction (predominantly flexibility) and problems with attention dominate. However, also memory deficits are described [30]. In detailed observation of single tasks aspects, e.g. in recalls of wordlists, primacy more than recency effects are shown, and recall is generally better.

While demented patients guess more often and describe things, depressed patients react with omissions and hesitant answers. Orientation is widely intact and confabulation, aphasic and apractic elements don't occur [22, 31].

3.2. The neuropsychological examination

Major tasks and aims of a neuropsychological examination comprise 1) determination and quantification of impaired cognitive function and resources as well as their consequences for maintaining all-day life, 2) assessment on changes of cognitive dysfunctions in progressive or reversible disease conditions, 3) differential diagnosis and securing of diagnosis as well as 4) evaluation of therapeutic benefits.

An important detail of the examination is a thorough interview with exploration of the clinical history, self-observation and observation of others, orientation, current mood situation (psychiatric side symptoms), as well as observation of behaviour during both interview and test situation. A final judgement is built from the test results with reference to emotional and motivational processes, a qualitative mistake analysis, and observation of behaviour during tests and interview, the resulting information derived from the interview and an evaluation of all-day competences during course of disease.

Neuropsychological testing represents an essential diagnostic tool in dementia diagnosis. It should be thoroughly performed and comprise the essential key competences. An "overtesting" should be avoided. In general, the choice of tests should orientate according to the individual differential diagnosis that is being questioned, the capacity of the individual patient and the time that is available.

Consecutively, a choice of test procedures is presented, that have been established in dementia diagnosis. As some of them cannot be administered solely for securing the diagnosis, a combination of several test procedures should be used.

For assessment of cognitive deficits in AD both screening methods as well as standardized psychometric tests are applied. Presumably, the most practical screening test in the clinical setting is the MMSE (Mini-Mental-State-Examination) according to Folstein et al. [32]. It comprises the examination of orientation in time and space, retentiveness and memory, attention and working memory, language (reading, writing, naming, speech comprehension, reading and meaning comprehension) as well as visual-spatial competences. The test takes usually approximately 10-12 minutes, the analysis results from a simple summation of points. At maximum 30 points can be achieved. The specificity ranges at 87 percent and the sensitivity at 82 percent [33]. However screening tests- as the mentioned MMSE- are only suitable, using cut off levels, for overviewing and determining severity of the dementia and for follow-up during disease course.

The MMSE is not acceptably sensitive in early onset dementia and does not allow, amongst other due to missing age and education correction, a satisfactory differentiation between "healthy" and "ill". For quantification of disease severity standard values of interpretation are provided, that can vary easily. Alternatively also CDR (Clinical Dementia Rating) or GDS (Global Deterioration Scale) can be applied. A general drop in points of around 3 MMSE points per year substantiates the suspected diagnosis of AD [34].

The *DemTect (Dementia Detection Test)*, likewise a screening test, focuses more precisely on Alzheimer-specific impairments with its task of word-list learning and delayed recall.

Furthermore it comprises more tasks on executive functions (working memory, word fluidity and cognitive flexibility). At maximum 18 points can be obtained. The DemTect is economic in time (8-12 minutes), it encloses a rough age correction (< 60 / ≥ 60 years) and presents with a high sensitivity for early stage AD and MCI [35].

After introduction in 1986 in the USA from the *Consortium to Establish a Registry for AD*, the newly established *CERAD test battery* has received great acceptance also in German-speaking countries. This novel neuropsychiatric testing tool has developed into a standardized dementia test procedure which aims to decipher cognitive dysfunction typical of AD [34, 36]. Analysed skills are: semantic fluidity (naming animals), naming of black and white drawings, verbal compliance and retentiveness (word list), delayed recall and recognition as well as constructive praxis (to copy something) and figural memory. The test battery also includes the MMSE. The results of a huge multicentre-validation study performed in German-speaking countries (n=1100), show that the variables: verbal fluidity, word list, memory, recall of wordlist, discrimination ability and recall of constructive praxis majorly contributed to the discriminability from healthy elderly persons to AD patients with a sensitivity of 87 percent and a specificity of 98 percent. Severe differences in profiles of AD patients, patients with vascular dementia and mixed dementia could not be obtained. A better discrimination was attained between AD patients, patients with depression and mild impairments. Both patients with depression and MCI ranged between Healthy and AD [36, 37].

To trace better on subcortical dysfunction, since 2005 additional tasks were included that aim to quantify on cognitive processing speed and flexibility (Trail making test A and B) as well as phonematic word fluidity tasks (words with initial letter "s") (CERAD-Plus). The whole test duration ranges between 30-45 minutes. The raw score are age- and education-matched (school and professional education) and also gender-matched. They are designated as z-levels as a measure of deviation to normal. The CERAD-Plus test battery allows a qualitative assessment on cognitive ability, on evaluation of disease severity and a follow up on repeated testing.

However, at present a parallel test version is not available, thus it is recommended to use an alternative test for memorising word lists when test intervals are on short-term. In suspicion of other underlying dementia causes further psychometric tests can be applied.

As an additional screening instrument for calculation of disease severity and for follow-up, the *clock-drawing test* is often recommended [38]. Next to visual-spatial abilities the test requires abilities in planning and semantic memory. The assessment includes, e.g. the integrity of the clock face, the presence of the clock hands, problems of drawing and conceptual difficulties. The sensitivity accounts for 90 percent, the specificity ranges at 56 percent. A qualitative evaluation is reasonable as well as the observation while drawing the clock face. In a qualitative feature analysis for securing the AD diagnosis in differentiation to patients with depression and healthy subjects (n=205, patients of a memory clinic) only errors occurred solely in patients with AD (with exception of one): in disorganised stereograms, only one clock-hand, mixing of numbers (1-12 with 12-24), mixing of minutes- and clock-hands, false or altered order of numbers and inability to write numbers [39].

In mind of the low specificity of the clock drawing test, Schmidtke et al. suggest an additional *clock reading test* with respect that it doesn't require higher executive function. The clock reading test is culture-, language-, education- and gender-independent, however shows a slight age-effect. It is easy to use and quickly analysable by a simple point system. Both in AD and LBD abnormalities are detected early and in comparison to healthy persons the sensitivity ranges at 82 percent, the specificity at 70 percent [24, 25].

In suspicion of an *apractic dysfunction*, a corresponding examination is informally possible, while allowing the patient to mimic easy gestures or mimic using distinct utensils (e.g. hammer, saw and scissors). As long as the patient is unable to perform the movements according to verbal request, one should allow him (to exclude problems with language comprehension) to imitate the demanded movements. For assessment of an ideatoric apraxia the patient is asked, e.g. to prepare a letter for shipment.

In order to examine *all-day competences* there are different tests available, e.g. the ADL-/ IADL-scale (Activities of Daily Living /Instrumental Activities of Daily Living), the Bayer-ADL-scale (Bayer Activities of Daily Living) or the FAQ (Functional Activities Questionnaire) which evaluate distinct functions partially very detailed. These tests are completed in general by relatives or by the interviewer [40-42]. Hereby, the FAQ has proven more sensitive compared to the IADL (85% to 57%) in the differentiation of "demented" and "normal". The specificity ranged at 81 percent [42].

Psychiatric side symptoms, e.g. *depression*, are assessed early during the neuropsychiatric interview. As needed additional depression scales can be used, e.g. the Geriatric Depression scale (GDS) or the Beck Depression Inventar (BDI), that are available also in short profile [43]. The input of depression scales depends on each situation and on the cognitive capacity of the patient. It should not lead to extend the usual time of the whole neuropsychiatric test situation.

4. Diagnostic imaging methods in AD

4.1. Computerized Tomography (CT)

Computerized Tomography (CT) is helpful in the detection of atrophy as well as other focal processes in brain and spinal cord, however it is not sufficient to substantiate AD diagnosis. Based on the low tissue contrast in comparison to magnetic resonance imgaging (MRI), CT serves well in the diagnostic classification of dementia syndromes. Advantages compared to MRI include a shorter time of investigation, low costs and a broad distribution [44]. In addition, CT allows an uncomplicated monitoring of critically ill patients.

With progressing age, brain volume decreases due to dying neurons and decline in water content. The annual atrophy rate ranges at around 0.24 % of total brain volume and is visible by the expansion of the ventricular system [45].

In AD, patients show a progressive brain atrophy in advancing disease which lies above the age matched population. This is demonstrated by enlargement of sulci and a dilatation of the ventricular system. Hereby, the dilatation of the ventricular system points to a subcortical tissue loss whereas the enlargement of the outer CSF interspaces points to cortical tissue loss [46]. The senso-motoric and the primary-visual cortex stay unaffected.

4.2. Magnetic Resonance Imaging (MRI)

MRI allows a high-contrast presentation of neuro-anatomical structures, pathological processes as well as of functional changes in brain activity. With progressive age a higher exchange rate of fluids exists between the ventricular system and the brain parenchyma. This is visible in T2- and Fluid-attenuated inversion recovery (FLAIR)-sequences by signal alterations in the ependyma of the anterior horns [47]. Intermittent, subcortical and central signal increases in the white matter (white-matter-lesions) increase with progressive age. Additionally brain iron accumulation can be detected in basal ganglia by increasing signal changes in T2-sequences.

Already in early AD stages MRI can display brain atrophy patterns. These can predominamtly be located in the medial temporal lobe, in the hippocampus and the gyrus parahippocampalis. Also, the entorhinal cortex, the amygdala, basal ganglia as well as thalamus and the parietal cortex can be involved [44]. An important role in the early detection of AD plays the Nucleus basalis Meynert. The voxel-based morphometry (VBM) reduces the weaknesses of predominantly investigator-dependent manual volumetry [48]. Modern computer techniques allow the spatial recognition of specific brain regions or the whole brain [49]. Hereby the volume of the typically affected brain region is exactly displayed and is comparable to that of other control groups. The majority of published studies show that patients with a MCI present with a smaller hippocampal volume than healthy controls and patients with AD have a smaller hippocampal volume in comparison to patients with MCI [50]. Patients with MCI hold an elevated risk for the development of AD [51]. Typical AD changes can also occur after brain trauma and long-lasting epilepsy.

Functional MRI (fMRI) has the potential to demonstrate cerebral blood flow as well as oxygen use of certain brain areas in response to specific stimuli or while processing certain cognitive tasks.

Due to the inherent magnetic properties of blood, represented by hemoglobin and deoxyhemoglobin, different patterns of activation are visible [44].

Despite of the high spatial resolution, this method presents with a high sensitivity for minor head movements. Studies of AD patients show a decrease of activitiy in the hippocampus, the parahippocampal areas as well as in the parietal and pre-frontal cortex in comparison to healthy control groups. Furthermore, fMRI is useful in monitoring of medical treatment in AD patients.

4.3. Emission computed tomography (SPECT and PET)

Imaging via single photon emission computed tomography (SPECT) and positron emission computed tomography (PET) allows the detection of local hemodynamic and metabolic dysfunction. After intravenous injection of a radioactive tracer and uptake in brain, the tracer localizes at the region of regional acitivity and images are taken. As the tracers often have short radioactive half life, the radioactive decay (emission of positrons) can be measured.

SPECT imaging shows the regional cerebral blood flow (rCBF) at rest by the regional uptake of glucose as an expression of neuronal activity. Hereby functional abnormalities can already be detected before symptom onset. The tracers ^{99m}Tc-HMPAO and ^{99m}Tc-ECD are mostly used in clinical practise. Due to their lipophilic character the tracers reach the cells in the first minutes after injection proportionately to rCBF [52]. The typical SPECT image in AD is characterized by a reduced rCBF in the medial and superior temporal lobes as well as in the posterior cingulum and precuneus without a reduced striatal DAT-binding [53]. Due to a very low spatial resolution of SPECT the diagnostic accuracy is lower than PET [54]. However application can be meaningful in clinical practise in order to differentiate other dementia causes.

PET imaging illustatrates a regional dysfunction of glucose metabolism via application of ^{18}F-FDG. Patients with AD demonstrate here, according to SPECT, a typical nuclide-distribution pattern of neuronal loss. Over 85 % of PET diagnosed AD patients could be neuropathologically verified [53]. At early AD disease stage and before symptom onset, a temporoparietal metabolic dysfunction is visible by voxel-based (volumetric pixel) analysis. Also patients with a genetic risk for development of AD show early decreases in signal activity [55]. As PET is the most efficient method for diagnostic verification of an AD, it has meanwhile established to a standard tool in dementia research [56].

For further diagnostic approaches the tracer ^{11}C-PIB was developed, which allows detection and distribution of Aß-plaques *in vivo* [57]. Next to an efficient diagnostic procedure and early disease recognition the dimension of AD dementia can be illustrated.

5. Biomarkers in peripheral tissues

Biomarkers are used as indicators of normal and pathogenic processes in a broad range of tissues, especially in peripheral tissues, which facilitates the accessibility of testing samples with minimal invasive methods. Despite substantial progress has been made in the area of biomarker development to confirm the diagnosis at early-clinical AD stages, less is known about the potential role of biomarkers in peripheral tissues in the prediction of AD [58]. Since it has been demonstrated for decades the existence of biochemical changes in the brain preceding the clinical AD onset (up to 20 years in advance) [59, 60] it is suggested that these changes may be also indirectly reflected in biological fluids. However, no tests are currently available to confirm an early AD diagnosis prior to clinical or symptomatic manifestations. The ongoing standardization efforts and quality control programs in biomarkers analysis, the development of tests in fully automated instruments, the combined detection of the well-established core biomarkers, the discovery of new regulated molecules improving current sensibility and sensitivity and the analysis of novel promising biomarkers in large independent cohorts will boost biomarker´s performance and facilitate the introduction of new AD diagnosis and prognosis tests in biological fluids in clinical routine.

5.1. CSF

CSF is the prime target among biological fluids in the search of specific biomarkers related to neurological disorders. The easy accessibility to this biofluid and its singular biophysic-chemical characteristics make CSF ideal for biomarkers investigation. On one hand, CSF is not a very complex fluid, being composed of a restricted amount of metabolites [61], which facilitates technical screening for regulated molecules. On the other hand, the direct contact between CSF and the extracellular space of the brain puts CSF in a valuable position to be considered as a potential indicator of the pathological processes occurring in the brain during different disease stages. This last aspect has not been analysed in depth since real comparisons and correlations are cumbersome and can only be formally made when using CSF and brain tissues from the same patients and the same disease stages.

The performance of CSF biomarkers as a diagnostic tool has greatly improved in parallel with the improvement of detection methodologies such as new generation proteomic technologies and high-throughput transcriptomic methodologies (deep-sequencing, microarrays and quantitative PCR panels), which eased and expanded the possibilities to measure full expression signature in a single assay enabling the inference of networks and biological functions associated to deregulated datasets. Indeed, current data indicate the existence of deregulated levels of proteins, peptides, small RNAs, mitochondrial DNA and a broad range of metabolites in the CSF of AD samples. In addition new outcomes are expected from worldwide undergoing large longitudinal studies in very-well defined cohorts [62].

5.1.1. Protein biomarkers

In recent years, a number of reports have exploited proteomic techniques to study the levels of selected proteins and peptides in the CSF of healthy and diseased individuals. Current data indicate that proteins and peptides such as β-amyloid (Aβ1-42/Aβ42 and Aβ1-40/Aβ40), total tau and phosphorylated tau (p-tau) meet the criteria to discriminate AD from individuals suffering from other types of dementias, as well as from healthy individuals and are considered as the core AD biomarkers [63]. According to different studies these biomarkers meet the consensus recommendations on AD biomarkers that should have >80% sensitivity and >80% specificity [64]. Importantly, core AD biomarkers molecules correlate with neuropathological hallmarks of AD, such as the presence of extracellular amyloid plaques (Aβ peptides), axonal degeneration (tau protein) and neuronal tangles (p-tau).

Three main observations unveil the clinical relevance of these molecules. Firstly, their appropriate sensibility and sensitivity have been successfully validated by independent large-scale multicentre studies [65-69], although these studies also point out that biomarkers measurements present significant inter-laboratory variations [70]. Secondly, Aβ42, tau and p-tau have been validated as predictors of AD in patients with MCI [71-74]. Lastly, longitudinal studies indicate that, at least, Tau and Aβ42 in CSF reflect the underlying disease state in early clinical and late stages of AD.

5.1.1.1. Aβ peptides

Aβ42 along with Aβ40 is secreted into the extracellular space and biological fluids, including CSF, as consequence of the proteolytic activity of proteinases on the Amyloid precursor protein (APP). Both peptides are found in senile plaques but their intracellular production, aggregation rates and proposed pathogenic functions are significantly distinct [75-77].

A consistent decrease in Aβ42 levels has been observed in the CSF of patients suffering from AD in several studies [78-80] but also in Subcortical White-matter Dementia (SWD) [81] and in Down Syndrome (DS) [82]. Reduced Aβ42 levels in AD are suggested to reflect either sequestration of Aβ42 in senile plaques, since Aβ42 CSF levels inversely correlate with the presence of senile plaques [83], or due to non-detectable Aβ42 oligomers in the assay, although alternative explanations may be plausible. In FTD, Aβ42 levels are significantly lower than in control samples, but higher than in AD cases [81, 84]. Aβ42 sensitivity and specificity in AD samples ranges from 78 to 100% (mean 85,6%) and from 67 to 100% (mean 88,5%), respectively [78]. A recent meta-analysis of 50 analytical studies indicates that CSF Aβ42 concentrations are significantly lower in AD when compared to MCI, FTD, PD and VaD but only moderately lower when compared to LBD [85].

Contrary to what is observed with Aβ42, Aβ40 and Aβ38 levels are not altered in the CSF of AD patients [79, 86, 87], but a significant decrease in Aβ40 levels is observed in FTLD when compared to AD and control cases [88]. In addition, Aβ40 levels, and more markedly Aβ38 levels, are decreased in FTD when compared to control samples [89].

A growing body of evidence suggests the superior performance of Aβ42/Aβ40 ratio when compared to Aβ42 alone using different analytic assays [79, 90, 91]. Importantly Aβ42/Aβ40 ratio is able to predict the conversion from MCI patients to AD when compared to cognitively stable MCI patients and MCI patients who developed other forms of dementia [79]. Aβ42/Aβ40 ratio is also able to discriminate better AD from VaD, LBD and non-AD dementia than Aβ42 alone and equally AD from FTD and non-AD dementia than the combination of Aβ42, p-tau and total tau [92]. Multiple studies also show an increased sensitivity and specificity in the use of Aβ ratio when compared to Aβ42/tau ratio, although the performance of combined biomarker analysis in AD diagnosis and prognosis is still a matter under discussion [93-96].

In addition to the regulated levels of monomeric Aβ species in the CSF of AD patients, encouraging observations have been reported in the potential diagnostic and prognostic role of BACE1, one of the main enzymes involved in the pathological cleave of the APP. Several independent observations indicate the presence of higher BACE1 levels and activity in the CSF of MCI and AD samples when compared to controls [97-100]. BACE1 activity is also increased in CJD samples [101] suggesting common pathological mechanisms among both diseases. Importantly, BACE1 correlate with classical AD biomarker's profile, brain atrophy in AD cases [102] and ApoE4 genotype [99], the latter being associated with an increased Aβ peptide *ex vivo* production [103]. In addition, specific BACE1 inhibitors dramatically reduce the presence of Aβ peptides in the CSF of AD patients [104] pointing out for a direct correlation between brain Aβ peptide processing and Aβ CSF levels.

5.1.1.2. Aβ oligomers

Recent studies demonstrated the presence of increased levels of Aβ oligomeric species in the CSF of AD patients when compared to controls using a broad range of methodological approaches [105-110]. Indeed, the analysis of individual Aβ oligomeric species is gaining experimental momentum due to their potential specific role in AD pathogenesis. Aβ40 oligomers levels are found to be increased in the CSF of AD patients at different disease severity stages, and a combined analysis of Aβ40 oligomers and monomeric Aβ42 greatly improved sensitivity and specificity to 95% and 90%, respectively [108]. Although the pathogenic role of Aβ40 in AD is still under discussion Aβ40 deposits have been reported both in control and AD brains [111, 112]. Aβ40-positive senile plaques with amyloid core are frequently associated with microglia in contrast to Aβ42-positive plaques [111], suggesting a role of microglia in the generation and aggregation of Aβ40 species in diseased brain. However, the different ability of Aβ fibrils and oligomers to react with microglia suggests a more complex scenario [113].

Aβ42 oligomers are increased in the CSF of AD patients [114] and the ratio of Aβ oligomers to Aβ42 is significantly elevated in AD patients [115]. Interestingly, the increased levels of Aβ42 oligomers in the CSF of MCI and AD samples may explain decreased levels of monomeric Aβ42. The recent development of the protein misfolding cyclic amplification assay (PMCA), based on the seeding activity of Aβ oligomers catalysing the polymerization of the monomeric Aβ, permits the discrimination of AD samples from other neurodegenerative non-degenerative neurological diseases with a sensitivity of 90% and specificity of 92% [109]. The use of Aβ-PMCA as a prognostic tool for detection of MCI still needs to be established. Importantly, detection of Aβ oligomers in the CSF is highly dependent on the native or disaggregated state of these oligomers [114, 116].

The finding that regulated levels of Aβ oligomer species are present in the CSF of AD patients' biofluids has a tremendous translational interest, since growing evidences indicate that soluble Aβ oligomers rather than aggregated Aβ plaques are more likely to be the main pathogenic agents of disease [117-119]. Consequently, preliminary data indicate that the analysis of Aβ oligomers, combined with levels of soluble Aβ peptides, may be relevant disease predictors and valuable tools for the analysis of AD progression.

5.1.1.3. Tau

The levels of total tau in the CSF, contrary to Aβ42 levels, increase with age [120]. Increments in tau levels have also been described in the CSF of AD and MCI patients in a broad range of several studies [121, 122] ranging from moderate to severe depending on the methodology and cohort used [78]. It is believed that deregulated tau may be reflecting the neuronal and axonal damage present in brain tissue and, as a consequence, the presence of increased tau levels is not a specific event for AD. Accordingly, transient tau increments have been also reported in acute stroke [123], and the most increased tau levels are observed in prion diseases such as in CJD, where massive neuronal cell death is present [124, 125]. Higher CSF tau is also associated with smaller brain volume in individuals with AD [126]. On the other hand, neurological diseases with minor neuronal loss and other dementias such as VaD, LBD and alcoholic dementia reflect minor or no significant changes in the levels of tau protein in the CSF, and tauopathies such as FTD also present inconsistent data [121, 127, 128].

A meta-analysis from different studies comparing tau levels in different dementia samples found that, although tau levels in AD are significantly increased when compared to controls, tau concentrations are moderately elevated in LBD, FTLD and VaD impeding a clear stratification between disease groups. Nevertheless, tau levels are useful to differentiate VaD from stroke [129] and, as expected, only CJD is characterized by extremely increased tau values, resulting in a sensitivity and specificity over 90% [130].

The improved performance of tau when analysed together with other AD biomarkers has been widely demonstrated [131, 132]. The combined use of Aβ42 and tau discriminates better between controls and AD and is very useful to predict MCI progression [69, 133]. A recent study also showed that decreased Aβ42 and increased tau levels are able to discriminate LBD from PD patients in spite of both being synucleopathies [134]. In the same line of evidences, combination of α-synuclein levels and Aβ42/tau ratios improves the diagnostic accuracy of PD [135].

A broad range of studies also demonstrated the helpfulness of the combined analysis of tau with non-AD core biomarkers. Assessment of tau and neuronal thread protein raises specificity and sensitivity for AD when compared to the individual analysis of both proteins [136]. Similarly, integrated analysis of tau and the regional cerebral blood flow in the posterior cingulate cortex discriminates MCI progressing to AD from non-progressive MCI [137]. The combined analysis of tau is also valuable for discriminating other diseases besides AD. As an example, the merged analysis of tau and midbrain-to-pons atrophy is reported to be useful for early identification of progressive supranuclear palsy (PSP), discriminating PSP cases from controls and patients suffering from corticobasal syndrome (CBS) and FTD [138].

5.1.1.4. Phospho-tau

Similarly to total tau, p-tau levels are increased in AD samples, although higher variability on its specificity and sensibility is reported when compared to the non-phosphorylated tau form [78, 127]. Several considerations should be done in this regard.

On one hand, the number of studies analysing p-tau levels is not as large as those performed for its non-phosphorylated form. In addition, sensitivity and sensibility may depend on the analysed phosphorylation site, although sensitivity for AD seems equal for at least the three main epitopes used in clinical diagnosis [139]. Importantly, results from a meta-analysis study indicate that tau phosphorylated at the Threonine 181 levels are able to discriminate AD from other dementias and MCI [140].

On the other hand, the utility of p-tau in the differential AD diagnosis against other neurodegenerative diseases is advantageous over total tau since p-tau levels reflect AD pathogenesis [141]. Indeed, p-tau levels in the CSF may reflect the levels of tau phosphorylation in AD brains. Tau is more increased in the CSF of sCJD patients than in AD, while p-tau is only modestly increased in sCJD [142]. In addition, tau levels are increased in neurological diseases such as in acute ischemic stroke, while p-tau levels remains unaltered [123]. Indeed, tau phosphorylation is physiologically regulated during several biological processes such as neuronal development, while tau levels usually remain more stable. Therefore, a direct correlation between total tau and p-tau levels cannot be established, and several lines of evidence indicate that p-tau levels are differently regulated, not only in AD, but also in other neurodegenerative diseases. In this regard, the main tau kinase, Glycogen synthase kinase 3 (GSK3) is assumed to be hyperactivated in AD brain, inducing pathogenic tau hyperphosphorylation, aggregation and formation of the intracellular NFTs. Although a direct correlation between GSK3 activity and tangle formation in AD is still under discussion [143], GSK3 levels and activity are markedly reduced in sCJD brain [144]. Thus, the distinct regulation of tau phosphorylation in the brain of AD and CJD, may explain the different p-tau/tau ratios observed in both diseases, which permits a differential diagnosis [145].

Recently it has been observed that patients suffering from rpAD present highly increased p-tau levels in the CSF [146] when compared to controls and classical AD patients. Since it is estimated that rpAD may be accounting for 10-30% of all AD cases, it is urgently needed to establish if lack of disease stratification may lead to misinterpretation of p-tau analysis between rapidly progressive and classical AD forms. In this regard, a combination of high CSF tau without proportionally elevated p-tau-181 is associated with a faster rate of cognitive decline [147]. In this regard, longitudinal studies indicates that a combination of low Aβ42 and high tau and p-tau levels is highly predictive of MCI progression and cognitive decline rate [74, 148].

5.1.1.5. Inflammatory cytokines

A common feature in the Central Nervous System of neurodegenerative diseases is the presence of chronic neuroinflammation associated with an exacerbated gliosis [149]. The role of a chronic and sustained inflammation in neurodegeneration is still a matter of debate as neuroinflammation has been suggested to play both detrimental and protective functions depending on disease stage, brain region, activation of anti-inflammatory mechanisms and cellular milieu among others [150]. Besides these considerations point out a critical role of neuroinflammation in the molecular mechanisms linked to AD pathology [151] and a broad range of inflammatory cytokines and immune response mediators are increased in the CSF of AD patients. A correlation between inflammatory markers and biomarkers of neurodegeneration has been described [152], and consequently, neurodegenerative disorders with high inflammatory chronic profiles such as prion diseases [153] present higher inflammatory-related deregulations in the CSF [154, 155]. However, the specific inflammatory profile observed in different types of dementia and at different disease stages indicates that inflammatory biomarkers could be used as surrogate markers for AD diagnosis and prognosis.

The anti-inflammatory cytokine TGFβ–1 is consistently upregulated in AD cases [156, 157]. Interestingly, during the progression from MCI to AD, a pro-inflammatory state is proposed since MCI patients who progressed to AD showed higher TNFα and lower TGFβ–1 and Aβ42 levels than control individuals or those non progressing to AD [158]. These data are in agreement with increased levels of the acute-phase C-reactive protein (CRP) and IL-6 in the CSF of MCI patients when compared to AD patients, indicating that inflammatory mechanisms are already progressing even before changes in core AD biomarkers such as Aβ42 and tau can be detected in the CSF [159].

In relation to this, a comparative analysis between Amnestic Mild Cognitive Impairment (aMCI) and MS patients indicated that pro-inflammatory cytokines and CD45+ lymphocytes are present in the same levels in both diseases. Taking into account that MS can be considered the most representative neuroinflammatory disease, these observations indicate that inflammatory mechanisms may be crucial for AD etiopathology.

In this regard, the pro-inflammatory cytokine osteopontin (OPN), also known as the secreted phosphoprotein 1 (SPP1) and involved in macrophage recruitment to inflammatory sites and cytokine production [160], is also elevated in the CSF of AD patients and in MCI patients developing AD. OPN levels correlate with cognitive decline and with increased levels in early disease phases [161, 162]. OPN has also been found elevated in the CSF during attacks of MS [163].

In addition, the major acute-phase protein SAP (Serum amyloid P component) has lower levels in MCI patients who progressed to AD than in those who did not progress to AD [164], suggesting that low SAP levels are linked to an increased risk of progression to AD.

Alternative promising inflammatory-biomarkers have been proposed. On one hand, lipocalin 2, whose levels are decreased in the CSF of MCI and AD patients and increased in brain regions with associated AD pathology [165]. On the other hand, the astrocytic marker YKL-40, has been reported to be increased in AD at early stages of the disease [166-169] and in FTD and aMCI patients [166]. In addition YKL-40 levels correlate positively with the classical core biomarkers tau and p-tau [166].

5.1.1.6. MicroRNAs

microRNAs (miRNA) are endogenous small non-coding RNAs (20-22 nucleotides) that are involved in post-transcriptional gene regulation by targeting mRNAs for cleavage or translational repression [170]. miRNAs have emerged as key regulators of various aspects of neuronal development and dysfunction. Deregulated small RNA signatures, especially miRNAs, have been observed in the brain of a broad range of neurodegenerative diseases such as AD, PD, HD or ALS [171, 172] and experimental evidences ascribe a functional role to miRNAs in the pathogenic molecular mechanisms leading to neurodegeneration [173-175]. With the advent of high-throughput technologies, full transcriptomic signatures can be provided not only from tissues, but also from samples with small amounts of starting material such as biological fluids and associated exosomes [176-178]. In this regard, more than 100 circulating miRNAs are deregulated in pathological conditions [179] and some of them have been proposed as potential biomarkers for disease diagnosis and prognosis, mainly in cancer and neurodegenerative diseases. Regarding the levels of circulating miRNAs in AD, several studies already reported changes when compared to control samples. A recent pilot study in two different cohorts showed that hsa-miR-27a-3p expression is reduced in the CSF of AD patients [180]. Decreased levels of this miRNA correlate with high tau and low Aβ amyloid levels. A second study analysed a selected group of miRNA candidates and observed that miRNAs 34a, 125b and

146a levels were significantly lower in the CSF of AD patients when compared to control cases, while the levels of the miRNAs 29a and 29b were significantly higher [181]. In an independent study low levels of miRNA-146a were also detected in the CSF of AD patients [182]. In this regard the expression of miRNA-146a is increased in AD [183] and CJD brains [184], in AD mice models [185] and in scrapie mice [184]. miRNA-146a expression in AD mice models also correlates with senile plaque density and synaptic pathology [185]. This miRNA is induced by the interleukin IL-1β, modulating the expression of IL-6 and the cyclooxygenase COX-2 and acting as a negative regulator of the astrocyte-mediated inflammatory response [186, 187]. In addition miRNA-146a negatively regulates TLR signalling to prevent exacerbated inflammation, thus, it seems to play a key role in the modulation of the neuropathology associated to chronic inflammation in neurodegenerative diseases. Whether the regulation of miRNAs in CSF is a consequence of neuronal cell damage or a modulated pathogenic response is still a matter of discussion.

In summary, all preliminary studies argue for the presence of deregulated levels of miRNAs in the CSF of AD patients with potential translational value. Exclusion of blood contamination effects, standardization of the assays, together with cross-disease and technical validation in larger cohorts need to be carried out to assess the potential role of miRNAs signatures as specific diagnostic and prognosis biomarker tool in AD and to define new diagnostic therapeutic opportunities related to the miRNA field.

5.1.1.7. Mitochondrial DNA

A pioneering study demonstrated that asymptomatic patients at risk of AD and symptomatic AD patients exhibit a significant decrease in the levels of circulating cell-free mtDNA in the CSF [188]. Data were generated by qPCR and digital droplet PCR and validated in an independent cohort of patients. Interestingly, this decrease is disease-specific, as mtDNA levels in the CSF of FTLD patients remain unchanged. Since decreased levels of mtDNA precede the appearance of the classical AD biomarkers such as Aβ42, mtDNA is an excellent potential preclinical AD biomarker. Further studies in larger cohorts including rpAD and CJD samples will determinate the clinical use of mtDNA analysis as a prognosis AD biomarker.

5.1.1.8. Metabolic profile

The use of analytic technologies such as Nuclear magnetic resonance and Liquid chromatography–mass spectrometry to analyse the metabolic signatures of biological fluids deserves special attention [189]. The metabolic profile in human CSF samples of AD patients and age-matched healthy controls unveils the presence of a significant presence of deregulated metabolites in AD cases [190]. Among them, higher corticols levels are found in AD cases, which correlate with AD progression and severity. In addition, the same study proved that combined analysis of different metabolites may increase sensitivity and specificity above 80%.

A second metabolic profile study identified the deregulated metabolic pathways in the CSF of MCI and AD patients [191]. The number of altered pathways increased with disease severity. Among them, Krebs cycle was significantly affected in MCI and cholesterol and sphingolipids transport was altered in AD. A high percentage of altered pathways in the CSF were also deregulated in plasma from the same individuals (30% in MCI and 60% in AD, respectively). Deregulated pathways performing the best disease discrimination were biosynthesis and metabolism of cortisone and prostaglandin 2.

Finally, a third study using metabolomics in the CSF of MCI and AD patients demonstrated the presence of elevated methionine (MET), 5-hydroxyindoleacetic acid (5-HIAA), vanillyl-mandelic acid, xanthosine and glutathione levels in AD patients and elevated 5-HIAA, MET, hypoxanthine and other metabolites in MCI patients when compared to healthy controls. Metabolite ratios revealed changes within tryptophan, MET and purine pathways [192], showing a partial overlap between MCI and AD.

Metabolomics is a promising tool for AD diagnosis indicating a slightly lower or similar performance when compared to classical AD biomarkers such as tau and Aβ42 depending on the study. Further analysis in large independent cohorts, technical updates as well as a combination of metabolic profiling with classical or alternative biomarkers will define the potential use of high throughput metabolic analysis in the AD diagnostic field. Besides, metabolite signatures may help to unveil the progression mechanisms and pathways leading to different dementia stages.

5.2. Blood

Despite the description of altered levels of several molecules in the blood levels of several molecules in the blood of AD patients as AD clinical biomarkers. Direct analysis in blood or blood-derived serum or plasma samples presents a broad range of advantages over CSF analysis. Blood extraction is minimally invasive and sample is easily collected, processed and stored over time. However, variations in the levels of blood metabolites may be reflecting a broad spectrum of changes not directly related to the neurodegenerative process. In addition, the dynamic range of the changes are lower than in CSF obtaining, most of the times, incon-sistent data. Additionally, contrary to CSF, blood is a very complex fluid composed of different types of metabolites and cell types that present significant oscillations in response to external factors not related to pathogenic events. The analysis of specific blood cells could be an alternative approach to link potential biomarkers levels with AD pathology, being a field under intense study.

5.2.1. Protein biomarkers

The core CSF AD biomarkers present minimal alterations in plasma. Aβ40 levels are higher in AD than in controls, although a high overlap is observed between groups. No changes have been observed for Aβ42, and Aβ40 and both Aβ40 and Aβ42 levels showed no association with cognitive decline [86]. Albeit some partial overlap between groups, tau levels in plasma are increased in AD when compared to control and MCI patients. Interestingly, tau levels cannot differentiate non-progressive from AD progressive MCI patients and there is a lack of correlation between CSF and plasma tau levels [193].

High-throughputs proteomic studies have tried to report the complex deregulated signatures between control and AD samples. A 2D-Mass spectrometry-based study detected a deregulated set of proteins in AD plasma complement factor H precursor and α-2-macroglobulin, which were validated and correlated with disease severity [194]. Independent multi-analyte profiling studies also demonstrated the presence of deregulated levels of proteins in MCI and AD samples when compared to controls both in serum and plasma. Among them some hits are related to AD pathogenesis such as the apoE [195, 196] as well as a broad range of inflammatory mediators [196, 197]. In an array-based ELISA study, 18 signalling proteins were able to distinguish AD from control samples with high accuracy (90%) and to predict MCI to AD progression [198], although the validation of this dataset has been ambiguous [199, 200]. The observation of a high variability between independent analyses indicates that further validations by independent methodologies in different cohorts need to be performed before resolving the clinical relevance of high-throughput blood-based analysis.

Alternative plasma biomarkers include the brain-reactive autoantibodies, present in sera irrespective of the presence of any pathology. This finding led to the analysis of the potential AD-specific autoantibody signature, which has been suggested to possess diagnostic value due to its ability to distinguish AD cases from controls, PD and breast cancer samples [201].

5.2.2. microRNAs

miRNA signature from CSF is only slightly more stable when compared to serum, suggesting that both biofluids are appropriate for the screening analysis of small RNAs [202]. Therefore, several studies addressed the potential deregulated miRNA signature in blood-derived AD samples. Using a microarray and qPCR validation approach the miR-125b, miR-23a and miR-26b were downregulated in the serum of AD cases when compared to non-inflammatory and inflammatory neurological controls and to FTD cases [203]. miR-125b presented the best accuracy discriminating AD from other groups. The same study observed that miR-125b and miR-26b levels were also diminished in the CSF of AD patients. An independent validation study was able to replicate downregulation of miR-125b in AD serum [204].

In a different approach, using RNA-sequencing and qPCR validation, downregulated levels of the miR-98-5p, miR-885-5p, miR-483-3p, miR-342-3p, miR-191-5p and let-7d-5p in the serum of AD cases were reported. The miR-342-3p showed the best sensitivity and specificity and correlated with cognitive decline [205]. However, downregulated levels of miR-342-3p in biological fluids are also a common hallmark in cancer [206]. Using a similar approach a 12 blood-based miRNA signatures was suggested to discriminate AD patients from controls and samples from patients suffering from different neurodegenerative diseases with high diagnostic accuracies [207]. Nonetheless, the different sample origin impedes a formal comparison between disease group's studies. The analysis of peripheral blood mononuclear cells identified upregulated levels of miR-34a, miR-181b in AD cells [208].

Despite the promising future of miRNA as biomarkers tools of clinical relevance, several considerations needs to be done. Lack of validation among current available studies, even when using similar platform, indicates that sample collection and methodology needs further standardization. In addition, high-throughput data need to be cross-validated in longitudinal studies using different cohorts and selected miRNAs validated in multicentre studies. Under these conditions miRNA in blood-related samples may serve as prognostic and diagnostic through the analysis of miRNA signatures alone or combined with the analysis of classical AD biomarkers.

6. Conclusion

The use of combined analysis of current AD diagnostic tools is gaining experimental momentum due to its demonstrated value as a better prognostic and diagnostic tool when compared to individual assessments. As most promising candidates, CSF markers as well as methods of in vivo neuroimaging have been identified. Among them, we can find structural MRI, ^{18}F-FDG-PET and novel in vivo amyloid-PET imaging [209, 210]. In longitudinal studies it was shown that with the help of these biomarkers AD could be diagnosed already in mild symptomatic states with high accuray allowing a predictability of its development [210]. Investigations of patients with genetic AD have demonstrated already 15 years prior to the onset of dementia significant pathological alterations in distinct biomarkers [211, 212].

Although these results are only assignable in a limited way to sporadic AD, the latter study provides impressive evidence on the long preclinical course of AD.

Current diagnostic concepts should therefore apply not at first when AD dementia has developed, but support explicitly the application of biomarkers at distinct stages of AD as it was shown that biomarkers become positive already at early and presymptomatic stages [213, 214].

In conclusion, differential diagnosis of a dementia syndrom requires esides clinical history and neuropsychological testing, analysis of metabolites in biological fluids as well as imaging methods. All these diagnostic approaches will not only allow an explanation towards the underlying cause of dementia but will also be useful in monitoring disease treatment and progression. The detection of AD at an early stage is hereby essential, as a further disease progression can be influenced positively by early initiation of treatment.

Integration of data generated during the last decades should be used to build up a worldwide rational algorithm based in the use of standardized, economically affordable methodologies and easily accessible samples.

Nomenclature

AD: Alzheimer's disease, rpAD: rapidly progressive Alzheimer's disease, CJD: Creutzfeldt-Jakob disease, aMCI: Amnestic Mild Cognitive Impairment, MCI: Mild cognitive impairment, FTLD: Frontotemporal Lobe Degeneration, FTD: Frontotemporal Dementia, CSF: Cerebrospinal Fluid, PD: Parkinson Disease, HD: Huntington Disease, ELISA: Enzyme-Linked Immuno-Sorbent Assay, MS: Multiple Sclerosis, SWD: Subcortical White-matter Dementia, MMSE: Mini–mental state examination, APP: Amyloid precursor protein, DS: Down Syndrome, CRP:

C-reactive protein, PSP: progressive supranuclear palsy, CBS: corticobasal syndrome; NINCDS/ADRDA: American National Institute of Neurological and Communicative Disorders and Stroke /Alzheimer's disease and Related Disorders Association; DGPPN: German Society of Psychiatry, Psychotherapy and Neurology; DGN: German Neurological Society; MRI: Magnetic Resonance Imaging, PET: Emission Computed Tomography; SPECT: single photon emission computed tomography; EEG: Electroencephalogram; CT; Computerized Tomography; CDR: Clinical Dementia Rating; GDS: Global Deterioration Scale; ADL-/IADL: Activities of Daily Living /Instrumental Activities of Daily Living; VBM: voxel-based morphometry; FLAIR; Fluid-attenuated inversion recovery; rCBF: regional cerebral blood flow.

Acknowledgements

The study was supported by the EU grants JPND-DEMTEST (Biomarker based diagnosis of rapid progressive dementias-optimization of diagnostic protocols, 01ED1201A) and PRIORITY (Protecting the food chain from prions, FP7-KBBE-2007-2A) and by funds from the Federal Ministry of Health (grant no. 1369-341] and from the German Center for Neurodegenerative Diseases (DZNE).

Author details

Franc Llorens[1,2], Sabine Nuhn[1], Christoph Peter[1], Inga Zerr[1,2] and Katharina Stoeck[1]

1 Department of Neurology, Clinical Dementia Center, University Medical School, Georg-August University, Göttingen, Germany

2 German Center for Neurodegenerative Diseases (DZNE) – Göttingen, Germany

References

[1] Hebert LE, Scherr PA, Bienias JL, Bennett DA, Evans DA. Alzheimer disease in the US population: prevalence estimates using the 2000 census. *Arch Neurol* 2003 Aug; 60:1119-1122.

[2] Brookmeyer R, Johnson E, Ziegler-Graham K, Arrighi HM. Forecasting the global burden of Alzheimer's disease. *Alzheimers Dement* 2007 Jul;3:186-191.

[3] Boise L, Neal MB, Kaye J. Dementia assessment in primary care: results from a study in three managed care systems. *J Gerontol A Biol Sci Med Sci* 2004 Jun;59:M621-M626.

[4] Boustani M, Peterson B, Hanson L, Harris R, Lohr KN. Screening for dementia in primary care: a summary of the evidence for the U.S. Preventive Services Task Force. *Ann Intern Med* 2003 Jun 3;138:927-937.

[5] Gaugler JE, Ascher-Svanum H, Roth DL, Fafowora T, Siderowf A, Beach TG. Characteristics of patients misdiagnosed with Alzheimer's disease and their medication use: an analysis of the NACC-UDS database. *BMC Geriatr* 2013;13:137.

[6] Komarova NL, Thalhauser CJ. High degree of heterogeneity in Alzheimer's disease progression patterns. *PLoS Comput Biol* 2011 Nov;7:e1002251.

[7] Koedam EL, Lauffer V, van der Vlies AE, van der Flier WM, Scheltens P, Pijnenburg YA. Early-versus late-onset Alzheimer's disease: more than age alone. *J Alzheimers Dis* 2010;19:1401-1408.

[8] Schmidt C, Redyk K, Meissner B, et al. Clinical features of rapidly progressive Alzheimer's disease. *Dement Geriatr Cogn Disord* 2010;29:371-378.

[9] de Leon MJ, Mosconi L, Blennow K, et al. Imaging and CSF studies in the preclinical diagnosis of Alzheimer's disease. *Ann N Y Acad Sci* 2007 Feb;1097:114-145.

[10] Walhovd KB, Fjell AM, Brewer J, et al. Combining MR imaging, positron-emission tomography, and CSF biomarkers in the diagnosis and prognosis of Alzheimer disease. *AJNR Am J Neuroradiol* 2010 Feb;31:347-354.

[11] Boutoleau-Bretonniere C, Lebouvier T, Delaroche O, et al. Value of neuropsychological testing, imaging, and CSF biomarkers for the differential diagnosis and prognosis of clinically ambiguous dementia. *J Alzheimers Dis* 2012;28:323-336.

[12] Shaffer JL, Petrella JR, Sheldon FC, et al. Predicting cognitive decline in subjects at risk for Alzheimer disease by using combined cerebrospinal fluid, MR imaging, and PET biomarkers. *Radiology* 2013 Feb;266:583-591.

[13] Edwards M, Balldin VH, Hall J, O'Bryant S. Combining Select Neuropsychological Assessment with Blood-Based Biomarkers to Detect Mild Alzheimer's Disease: A Molecular Neuropsychology Approach. *J Alzheimers Dis* 2014 Jun 10.

[14] Deutsche Gesellschaft für Psychiatrie PuNDDGfND. Demenzen. S3-Leitlinie, 2009.

[15] McKhann G, Drachman D, Folstein M, Katzman R, Price D, Stadlan EM. Clinical diagnosis of Alzheimer's disease: report of the NINCDS-ADRDA Work Group under the auspices of Department of Health and Human Services Task Force on Alzheimer's Disease. *Neurology* 1984 Jul;34:939-944.

[16] McKhann GM, Knopman DS, Chertkow H, et al. The diagnosis of dementia due to Alzheimer's disease: recommendations from the National Institute on Aging-Alzheimer's Association workgroups on diagnostic guidelines for Alzheimer's disease. *Alzheimers Dement* 2011 May;7:263-269.

[17] Dubois B, Feldman HH, Jacova C, et al. Research criteria for the diagnosis of Alzheimer's disease: revising the NINCDS-ADRDA criteria. *Lancet Neurol* 2007 Aug; 6:734-746.

[18] Albert MS, Dekosky ST, Dickson D, et al. The diagnosis of mild cognitive impairment due to Alzheimer's disease: recommendations from the National Institute on Aging-Alzheimer's Association workgroups on diagnostic guidelines for Alzheimer's disease. *Alzheimers Dement* 2011 May;7:270-279.

[19] Winblad B, Palmer K, Kivipelto M, et al. Mild cognitive impairment--beyond controversies, towards a consensus: report of the International Working Group on Mild Cognitive Impairment. *J Intern Med* 2004 Sep;256:240-246.

[20] Petersen RC. Clinical practice. Mild cognitive impairment. *N Engl J Med* 2011 Jun 9;364:2227-2234.

[21] Loewenstein D. Assessment of Alzheimer's Disease. Handbook on the Neuropsychology of Aging and Dementia. Springer, 2013:271-280.

[22] Jahn T. Neuropsychologie der Demenz. Lautenbacher S, Gauggel (Hrsg.): Neuropsychologie psychischer Störungen. Springer, 2010:360-381.

[23] Schmidtke K. Otto, M. Demenzen. Wallesch, CW, Förstl, H (Hrsg.) Thieme, 2012:203-227.

[24] Schmidtke K, Olbrich S. The Clock Reading Test: validation of an instrument for the diagnosis of dementia and disorders of visuo-spatial cognition. *Int Psychogeriatr* 2007 Apr;19:307-321.

[25] Schmidtke K. Neuropsychologische Untersuchung bei Patienten mit Demenzverdacht. In: Hüll M, ed., 26 ed Nervenheilkunde, 2007:651-658.

[26] Tsai PH, Teng E, Liu C, Mendez MF. Posterior cortical atrophy: evidence for discrete syndromes of early-onset Alzheimer's disease. *Am J Alzheimers Dis Other Demen* 2011 Aug;26:413-418.

[27] Groh-Bordin C. Störungen der Visuellen Raumwahrnehmung und Raumkognition. In: Kerkhoff G, ed. Sturm, W. et al. (Hrsg.): Lehrbuch der Klinischen Neuropsychologie, Springer, 2009:500-512.

[28] Monsch AU, Bondi MW, Butters N, Salmon DP, Katzman R, Thal LJ. Comparisons of verbal fluency tasks in the detection of dementia of the Alzheimer type. *Arch Neurol* 1992 Dec;49:1253-1258.

[29] Engel S. Kognitives Screening. In: Mück A LFR, ed. Demenzerkrankungen. Deutscher Ärzte-Verlag Mahlberg R, Gutzmann (Hrsg.). 2009.

[30] Beblo T. Neuropsychologie affektiver Störungen. Neuropsychologie psychischer Störungen. 2. Auflage Lautenbacher, S, Gauggel, S (Hrsg.). 2010:211-218.

[31]   Beblo T. Neuropsychologie der Depression. In: Lautenbacher S, ed. Göttingen: Hog-refe, 2006.

[32]   Folstein MF, Folstein SE, McHugh PR. "Mini-mental state". A practical method for grading the cognitive state of patients for the clinician. *J Psychiatr Res* 1975 Nov; 12:189-198.

[33]   Anthony JC, LeResche L, Niaz U, Von Korff MR, Folstein MF. Limits of the 'Mini-Mental State' as a screening test for dementia and delirium among hospital patients. *Psychol Med* 1982 May;12:397-408.

[34]   Ivemeyer D. Demenztests in der Praxis. In: Zerfaß R, ed. München: Urban & Fischer, 2006.

[35]   Kalbe E, Kessler J, Calabrese P, et al. DemTect: a new, sensitive cognitive screening test to support the diagnosis of mild cognitive impairment and early dementia. *Int J Geriatr Psychiatry* 2004 Feb;19:136-143.

[36]   Aebi C. Validierung der neuropsychologischen Testbatterie CERAD-NP. Eine Multi-Center Studie. Dissertation, Bassel 2002.: 2002.

[37]   Barth S. Neuropsychologische Profile in der Demenzdiagnostik: Eine Untersuchung mit der CERAD-NP-Testbatterie. In: Schönknecht PPJSJ, ed. Fortschritte Neurologie Psychiatrie : 2005:1-9.

[38]   Shulman KI. Clock-drawing: is it the ideal cognitive screening test? *Int J Geriatr Psychiatry* 2000 Jun;15:548-561.

[39]   Schröder MR et al. Merkmalsanalyse von Uhrzeichnungen als Beitrag zur Diagnostik der Demenz vom Alzheimer Typ. In: Hasse-Sander IMHHRMHJ, ed., 12 ed Zeitschrift für Gerontopsychologie & -psychiatrie, 1999:55-66.

[40]   Lawton MP, Brody EM. Assessment of older people: self-maintaining and instrumental activities of daily living. *Gerontologist* 1969;9:179-186.

[41]   Erzigkeit H, Lehfeld H, Pena-Casanova J, et al. The Bayer-Activities of Daily Living Scale (B-ADL): results from a validation study in three European countries. *Dement Geriatr Cogn Disord* 2001 Sep;12:348-358.

[42]   Pfeffer RI, Kurosaki TT, Harrah CH, Jr., Chance JM, Filos S. Measurement of functional activities in older adults in the community. *J Gerontol* 1982 May;37:323-329.

[43]   Yesavage JA, Brink TL, Rose TL, et al. Development and validation of a geriatric depression screening scale: a preliminary report. *J Psychiatr Res* 1982;17:37-49.

[44]   Ortiz-Teran L. Currently Available Neuroimaging Approaches in Alzheimer Disease (AD) Early Diagnosis. In: et al, ed. Suzanne de La Monte (Hg.): The Clinical Spectrum of Alzheimer's Disease -The Charge Toward Comprehensive Diagnostic and Therapeutic Strategies: InTech., 2011.

[45] de Leon MJ, George AE, Golomb J, et al. Frequency of hippocampal formation atrophy in normal aging and Alzheimer's disease. *Neurobiol Aging* 1997 Jan;18:1-11.

[46] Wallesch C. Demenzen. 2., überarbeitete und erweiterte Auflage. Stuttgart: Thieme (Referenzreihe Neurologie Herausgegeben von G. Deuschl, H.C. Diener, H.C. Hopf)., 2012.

[47] Reiser M. Radiologie. 3., vollst. überarb. u. erw. Aufl. In: et al, ed. Stuttgart: Thieme (Duale Reihe)., 2011.

[48] Kinkingnehun S, Sarazin M, Lehericy S, Guichart-Gomez E, Hergueta T, Dubois B. VBM anticipates the rate of progression of Alzheimer disease: a 3-year longitudinal study. *Neurology* 2008 Jun 3;70:2201-2211.

[49] Thompson PM, Hayashi KM, de Zubicaray GI, et al. Mapping hippocampal and ventricular change in Alzheimer disease. *Neuroimage* 2004 Aug;22:1754-1766.

[50] Becker JT, Davis SW, Hayashi KM, et al. Three-dimensional patterns of hippocampal atrophy in mild cognitive impairment. *Arch Neurol* 2006 Jan;63:97-101.

[51] Apostolova LG, Steiner CA, Akopyan GG, et al. Three-dimensional gray matter atrophy mapping in mild cognitive impairment and mild Alzheimer disease. *Arch Neurol* 2007 Oct;64:1489-1495.

[52] Farid K, Caillat-Vigneron N, Sibon I. Is brain SPECT useful in degenerative dementia diagnosis? *J Comput Assist Tomogr* 2011 Jan;35:1-3.

[53] Mosconi L, Berti V, Glodzik L, Pupi A, De SS, de Leon MJ. Pre-clinical detection of Alzheimer's disease using FDG-PET, with or without amyloid imaging. *J Alzheimers Dis* 2010;20:843-854.

[54] Matsuda H. Cerebral blood flow and metabolic abnormalities in Alzheimer's disease. *Ann Nucl Med* 2001 Apr;15:85-92.

[55] Duran FL, Zampieri FG, Bottino CC, Buchpiguel CA, Busatto GF. Voxel-based investigations of regional cerebral blood flow abnormalities in Alzheimer's disease using a single-detector SPECT system. *Clinics (Sao Paulo)* 2007 Aug;62:377-384.

[56] Herholz K, Carter SF, Jones M. Positron emission tomography imaging in dementia. *Br J Radiol* 2007 Dec;80 Spec No 2:S160-S167.

[57] Morris JC, Roe CM, Grant EA, et al. Pittsburgh compound B imaging and prediction of progression from cognitive normality to symptomatic Alzheimer disease. *Arch Neurol* 2009 Dec;66:1469-1475.

[58] Blennow K, Zetterberg H, Fagan AM. Fluid biomarkers in Alzheimer disease. *Cold Spring Harb Perspect Med* 2012 Sep;2:a006221.

[59] Price JL, Morris JC. Tangles and plaques in nondemented aging and "preclinical" Alzheimer's disease. *Ann Neurol* 1999 Mar;45:358-368.

[60] Davies L, Wolska B, Hilbich C, et al. A4 amyloid protein deposition and the diagnosis of Alzheimer's disease: prevalence in aged brains determined by immunocytochemistry compared with conventional neuropathologic techniques. *Neurology* 1988 Nov;38:1688-1693.

[61] Cutler RW, Spertell RB. Cerebrospinal fluid: a selective review. *Ann Neurol* 1982 Jan; 11:1-10.

[62] Fagan AM. CSF Biomarkers of Alzheimer's Disease: Impact on Disease Concept, Diagnosis, and Clinical Trial Design. Advances in Geriatry 2014.

[63] Blennow K, Hampel H, Weiner M, Zetterberg H. Cerebrospinal fluid and plasma biomarkers in Alzheimer disease. *Nat Rev Neurol* 2010 Mar;6:131-144.

[64] Consensus report of the Working Group on: "Molecular and Biochemical Markers of Alzheimer's Disease". The Ronald and Nancy Reagan Research Institute of the Alzheimer's Association and the National Institute on Aging Working Group. *Neurobiol Aging* 1998 Mar;19:109-116.

[65] Mattsson N, Zetterberg H, Hansson O, et al. CSF biomarkers and incipient Alzheimer disease in patients with mild cognitive impairment. *JAMA* 2009 Jul 22;302:385-393.

[66] Kanai M, Matsubara E, Isoe K, et al. Longitudinal study of cerebrospinal fluid levels of tau, A beta1-40, and A beta1-42(43) in Alzheimer's disease: a study in Japan. *Ann Neurol* 1998 Jul;44:17-26.

[67] Shoji M, Matsubara E, Murakami T, et al. Cerebrospinal fluid tau in dementia disorders: a large scale multicenter study by a Japanese study group. *Neurobiol Aging* 2002 May;23:363-370.

[68] Visser PJ, Verhey F, Knol DL, et al. Prevalence and prognostic value of CSF markers of Alzheimer's disease pathology in patients with subjective cognitive impairment or mild cognitive impairment in the DESCRIPA study: a prospective cohort study. *Lancet Neurol* 2009 Jul;8:619-627.

[69] Shaw LM, Vanderstichele H, Knapik-Czajka M, et al. Cerebrospinal fluid biomarker signature in Alzheimer's disease neuroimaging initiative subjects. *Ann Neurol* 2009 Apr;65:403-413.

[70] Mattsson N, Zetterberg H, Blennow K. Lessons from Multicenter Studies on CSF Biomarkers for Alzheimer's Disease. *Int J Alzheimers Dis* 2010;2010.

[71] Hampel H, Teipel SJ, Fuchsberger T, et al. Value of CSF beta-amyloid1-42 and tau as predictors of Alzheimer's disease in patients with mild cognitive impairment. *Mol Psychiatry* 2004 Jul;9:705-710.

[72] Herukka SK, Hallikainen M, Soininen H, Pirttila T. CSF Abeta42 and tau or phosphorylated tau and prediction of progressive mild cognitive impairment. *Neurology* 2005 Apr 12;64:1294-1297.

[73]   Hansson O, Zetterberg H, Buchhave P, Londos E, Blennow K, Minthon L. Associa-
       tion between CSF biomarkers and incipient Alzheimer's disease in patients with mild
       cognitive impairment: a follow-up study. *Lancet Neurol* 2006 Mar;5:228-234.

[74]   Snider BJ, Fagan AM, Roe C, et al. Cerebrospinal fluid biomarkers and rate of cogni-
       tive decline in very mild dementia of the Alzheimer type. *Arch Neurol* 2009 May;
       66:638-645.

[75]   Hartmann T, Bieger SC, Bruhl B, et al. Distinct sites of intracellular production for
       Alzheimer's disease A beta40/42 amyloid peptides. *Nat Med* 1997 Sep;3:1016-1020.

[76]   Hampel H, Shen Y, Walsh DM, et al. Biological markers of amyloid beta-related
       mechanisms in Alzheimer's disease. *Exp Neurol* 2010 Jun;223:334-346.

[77]   Hoshi M, Sato M, Matsumoto S, et al. Spherical aggregates of beta-amyloid (amylos-
       pheroid) show high neurotoxicity and activate tau protein kinase I/glycogen syn-
       thase kinase-3beta. *Proc Natl Acad Sci U S A* 2003 May 27;100:6370-6375.

[78]   Blennow K. Cerebrospinal fluid protein biomarkers for Alzheimer's disease. *NeuroRx*
       2004 Apr;1:213-225.

[79]   Hansson O, Zetterberg H, Buchhave P, et al. Prediction of Alzheimer's disease using
       the CSF Abeta42/Abeta40 ratio in patients with mild cognitive impairment. *Dement
       Geriatr Cogn Disord* 2007;23:316-320.

[80]   Vanmechelen E, Vanderstichele H, Hulstaert F, et al. Cerebrospinal fluid tau and be-
       ta-amyloid(1-42) in dementia disorders. *Mech Ageing Dev* 2001 Nov;122:2005-2011.

[81]   Sjogren M, Minthon L, Davidsson P, et al. CSF levels of tau, beta-amyloid(1-42) and
       GAP-43 in frontotemporal dementia, other types of dementia and normal aging. *J
       Neural Transm* 2000;107:563-579.

[82]   Tamaoka A, Sekijima Y, Matsuno S, Tokuda T, Shoji S, Ikeda SI. Amyloid beta pro-
       tein species in cerebrospinal fluid and in brain from patients with Down's syndrome.
       Ann Neurol 1999 Dec;46:933.

[83]   Strozyk D, Blennow K, White LR, Launer LJ. CSF Abeta 42 levels correlate with amy-
       loid-neuropathology in a population-based autopsy study. *Neurology* 2003 Feb
       25;60:652-656.

[84]   Riemenschneider M, Wagenpfeil S, Diehl J, et al. Tau and Abeta42 protein in CSF of
       patients with frontotemporal degeneration. *Neurology* 2002 Jun 11;58:1622-1628.

[85]   Tang W, Huang Q, Wang Y, Wang ZY, Yao YY. Assessment of CSF Abeta as an aid to
       discriminating Alzheimer's disease from other dementias and mild cognitive impair-
       ment: A meta-analysis of 50 studies. *J Neurol Sci* 2014 Jul 15.

[86]   Mehta PD, Pirttila T, Mehta SP, Sersen EA, Aisen PS, Wisniewski HM. Plasma and
       cerebrospinal fluid levels of amyloid beta proteins 1-40 and 1-42 in Alzheimer dis-
       ease. *Arch Neurol* 2000 Jan;57:100-105.

[87] Schoonenboom NS, Mulder C, Van Kamp GJ, et al. Amyloid beta 38, 40, and 42 species in cerebrospinal fluid: more of the same? *Ann Neurol* 2005 Jul;58:139-142.

[88] Pijnenburg YA, Schoonenboom SN, Mehta PD, et al. Decreased cerebrospinal fluid amyloid beta (1-40) levels in frontotemporal lobar degeneration. *J Neurol Neurosurg Psychiatry* 2007 Jul;78:735-737.

[89] Gabelle A, Roche S, Geny C, et al. Decreased sAbetaPPbeta, Abeta38, and Abeta40 cerebrospinal fluid levels in frontotemporal dementia. *J Alzheimers Dis* 2011;26:553-563.

[90] Lewczuk P, Lelental N, Spitzer P, Maler JM, Kornhuber J. Amyloid-beta 42/40 Cerebrospinal Fluid Concentration Ratio in the Diagnostics of Alzheimer's Disease: Validation of Two Novel Assays. *J Alzheimers Dis* 2014 Jul 30.

[91] Shoji M, Matsubara E, Kanai M, et al. Combination assay of CSF tau, A beta 1-40 and A beta 1-42(43) as a biochemical marker of Alzheimer's disease. *J Neurol Sci* 1998 Jun 30;158:134-140.

[92] Spies PE, Slats D, Sjogren JM, et al. The cerebrospinal fluid amyloid beta42/40 ratio in the differentiation of Alzheimer's disease from non-Alzheimer's dementia. *Curr Alzheimer Res* 2010 Aug;7:470-476.

[93] Wiltfang J, Esselmann H, Bibl M, et al. Amyloid beta peptide ratio 42/40 but not A beta 42 correlates with phospho-Tau in patients with low- and high-CSF A beta 40 load. *J Neurochem* 2007 May;101:1053-1059.

[94] Lewczuk P, Esselmann H, Otto M, et al. Neurochemical diagnosis of Alzheimer's dementia by CSF Abeta42, Abeta42/Abeta40 ratio and total tau. *Neurobiol Aging* 2004 Mar;25:273-281.

[95] Bombois S, Duhamel A, Salleron J, et al. A new decision tree combining Abeta 1-42 and p-Tau levels in Alzheimer's diagnosis. *Curr Alzheimer Res* 2013 May 1;10:357-364.

[96] Parnetti L, Chiasserini D, Eusebi P, et al. Performance of abeta1-40, abeta1-42, total tau, and phosphorylated tau as predictors of dementia in a cohort of patients with mild cognitive impairment. *J Alzheimers Dis* 2012;29:229-238.

[97] Holsinger RM, McLean CA, Collins SJ, Masters CL, Evin G. Increased beta-Secretase activity in cerebrospinal fluid of Alzheimer's disease subjects. *Ann Neurol* 2004 Jun; 55:898-899.

[98] Zhong Z, Ewers M, Teipel S, et al. Levels of beta-secretase (BACE1) in cerebrospinal fluid as a predictor of risk in mild cognitive impairment. *Arch Gen Psychiatry* 2007 Jun;64:718-726.

[99] Ewers M, Zhong Z, Burger K, et al. Increased CSF-BACE 1 activity is associated with ApoE-epsilon 4 genotype in subjects with mild cognitive impairment and Alzheimer's disease. *Brain* 2008 May;131:1252-1258.

[100] Zetterberg H, Andreasson U, Hansson O, et al. Elevated cerebrospinal fluid BACE1 activity in incipient Alzheimer disease. *Arch Neurol* 2008 Aug;65:1102-1107.

[101] Holsinger RM, Lee JS, Boyd A, Masters CL, Collins SJ. CSF BACE1 activity is increased in CJD and Alzheimer disease versus (corrected) other dementias. *Neurology* 2006 Aug 22;67:710-712.

[102] Ewers M, Cheng X, Zhong Z, et al. Increased CSF-BACE1 activity associated with decreased hippocampus volume in Alzheimer's disease. *J Alzheimers Dis* 2011;25:373-381.

[103] Ye S, Huang Y, Mullendorff K, et al. Apolipoprotein (apo) E4 enhances amyloid beta peptide production in cultured neuronal cells: apoE structure as a potential therapeutic target. *Proc Natl Acad Sci U S A* 2005 Dec 20;102:18700-18705.

[104] Menting KW, Claassen JA. beta-secretase inhibitor; a promising novel therapeutic drug in Alzheimer's disease. *Front Aging Neurosci* 2014;6:165.

[105] Fukumoto H, Tokuda T, Kasai T, et al. High-molecular-weight beta-amyloid oligomers are elevated in cerebrospinal fluid of Alzheimer patients. *FASEB J* 2010 Aug; 24:2716-2726.

[106] Santos AN, Ewers M, Minthon L, et al. Amyloid-beta oligomers in cerebrospinal fluid are associated with cognitive decline in patients with Alzheimer's disease. *J Alzheimers Dis* 2012;29:171-176.

[107] Holtta M, Hansson O, Andreasson U, et al. Evaluating amyloid-beta oligomers in cerebrospinal fluid as a biomarker for Alzheimer's disease. *PLoS One* 2013;8:e66381.

[108] Gao CM, Yam AY, Wang X, et al. Abeta40 oligomers identified as a potential biomarker for the diagnosis of Alzheimer's disease. *PLoS One* 2010;5:e15725.

[109] Salvadores N, Shahnawaz M, Scarpini E, Tagliavini F, Soto C. Detection of misfolded Abeta oligomers for sensitive biochemical diagnosis of Alzheimer's disease. *Cell Rep* 2014 Apr 10;7:261-268.

[110] Pitschke M, Prior R, Haupt M, Riesner D. Detection of single amyloid beta-protein aggregates in the cerebrospinal fluid of Alzheimer's patients by fluorescence correlation spectroscopy. *Nat Med* 1998 Jul;4:832-834.

[111] Fukumoto H, Asami-Odaka A, Suzuki N, Iwatsubo T. Association of A beta 40-positive senile plaques with microglial cells in the brains of patients with Alzheimer's disease and in non-demented aged individuals. *Neurodegeneration* 1996 Mar;5:13-17.

[112] Gravina SA, Ho L, Eckman CB, et al. Amyloid beta protein (A beta) in Alzheimer's disease brain. Biochemical and immunocytochemical analysis with antibodies specific for forms ending at A beta 40 or A beta 42(43). *J Biol Chem* 1995 Mar 31;270:7013-7016.

[113] Ferrera D, Mazzaro N, Canale C, Gasparini L. Resting microglia react to Abeta42 fibrils but do not detect oligomers or oligomer-induced neuronal damage. *Neurobiol Aging* 2014 May 29.

[114] Englund H, Degerman GM, Brundin RM, et al. Oligomerization partially explains the lowering of Abeta42 in Alzheimer's disease cerebrospinal fluid. *Neurodegener Dis* 2009;6:139-147.

[115] Herskovits AZ, Locascio JJ, Peskind ER, Li G, Hyman BT. A Luminex assay detects amyloid beta oligomers in Alzheimer's disease cerebrospinal fluid. *PLoS One* 2013;8:e67898.

[116] Sancesario GM, Cencioni MT, Esposito Z, et al. The load of amyloid-beta oligomers is decreased in the cerebrospinal fluid of Alzheimer's disease patients. *J Alzheimers Dis* 2012;31:865-878.

[117] Haass C, Selkoe DJ. Soluble protein oligomers in neurodegeneration: lessons from the Alzheimer's amyloid beta-peptide. *Nat Rev Mol Cell Biol* 2007 Feb;8:101-112.

[118] Shankar GM, Li S, Mehta TH, et al. Amyloid-beta protein dimers isolated directly from Alzheimer's brains impair synaptic plasticity and memory. *Nat Med* 2008 Aug; 14:837-842.

[119] Lesne S, Koh MT, Kotilinek L, et al. A specific amyloid-beta protein assembly in the brain impairs memory. *Nature* 2006 Mar 16;440:352-357.

[120] Sjogren M, Vanderstichele H, Agren H, et al. Tau and Abeta42 in cerebrospinal fluid from healthy adults 21-93 years of age: establishment of reference values. *Clin Chem* 2001 Oct;47:1776-1781.

[121] Humpel C. Identifying and validating biomarkers for Alzheimer's disease. *Trends Biotechnol* 2011 Jan;29:26-32.

[122] Andreasen N, Minthon L, Davidsson P, et al. Evaluation of CSF-tau and CSF-Abeta42 as diagnostic markers for Alzheimer disease in clinical practice. *Arch Neurol* 2001 Mar;58:373-379.

[123] Hesse C, Rosengren L, Andreasen N, et al. Transient increase in total tau but not phospho-tau in human cerebrospinal fluid after acute stroke. *Neurosci Lett* 2001 Jan 19;297:187-190.

[124] Stoeck K, Sanchez-Juan P, Gawinecka J, et al. Cerebrospinal fluid biomarker supported diagnosis of Creutzfeldt-Jakob disease and rapid dementias: a longitudinal multicentre study over 10 years. *Brain* 2012 Oct;135:3051-3061.

[125] Buerger K, Otto M, Teipel SJ, et al. Dissociation between CSF total tau and tau protein phosphorylated at threonine 231 in Creutzfeldt-Jakob disease. *Neurobiol Aging* 2006 Jan;27:10-15.

[126] Fagan AM, Head D, Shah AR, et al. Decreased cerebrospinal fluid Abeta(42) corre-lates with brain atrophy in cognitively normal elderly. *Ann Neurol* 2009 Feb; 65:176-183.

[127] Zetterberg H, Blennow K, Hanse E. Amyloid beta and APP as biomarkers for Alz-heimer's disease. *Exp Gerontol* 2010 Jan;45:23-29.

[128] Andreasen N, Vanmechelen E, Van d, V, et al. Cerebrospinal fluid tau protein as a biochemical marker for Alzheimer's disease: a community based follow up study. *J Neurol Neurosurg Psychiatry* 1998 Mar;64:298-305.

[129] Kaerst L, Kuhlmann A, Wedekind D, Stoeck K, Lange P, Zerr I. Cerebrospinal fluid biomarkers in Alzheimer's disease, vascular dementia and ischemic stroke patients: a critical analysis. *J Neurol* 2013 Nov;260:2722-2727.

[130] van Harten AC, Kester MI, Visser PJ, et al. Tau and p-tau as CSF biomarkers in de-mentia: a meta-analysis. *Clin Chem Lab Med* 2011 Mar;49:353-366.

[131] De R, V, Galloni E, Marcon M, et al. Analysis of combined CSF biomarkers in AD di-agnosis. *Clin Lab* 2014;60:629-634.

[132] Holtzman DM. CSF biomarkers for Alzheimer's disease: current utility and potential future use. *Neurobiol Aging* 2011 Dec;32 Suppl 1:S4-S9.

[133] Sunderland T, Linker G, Mirza N, et al. Decreased beta-amyloid1-42 and increased tau levels in cerebrospinal fluid of patients with Alzheimer disease. *JAMA* 2003 Apr 23;289:2094-2103.

[134] Kaerst L, Kuhlmann A, Wedekind D, Stoeck K, Lange P, Zerr I. Using cerebrospinal fluid marker profiles in clinical diagnosis of dementia with Lewy bodies, Parkinson's disease, and Alzheimer's disease. *J Alzheimers Dis* 2014;38:63-73.

[135] Parnetti L, Farotti L, Eusebi P, et al. Differential role of CSF alpha-synuclein species, tau, and Abeta42 in Parkinson's Disease. *Front Aging Neurosci* 2014;6:53.

[136] Kahle PJ, Jakowec M, Teipel SJ, et al. Combined assessment of tau and neuronal thread protein in Alzheimer's disease CSF. *Neurology* 2000 Apr 11;54:1498-1504.

[137] Okamura N, Arai H, Maruyama M, et al. Combined Analysis of CSF Tau Levels and ((123)I)Iodoamphetamine SPECT in Mild Cognitive Impairment: Implications for a Novel Predictor of Alzheimer's Disease. *Am J Psychiatry* 2002 Mar;159:474-476.

[138] Borroni B, Malinverno M, Gardoni F, et al. A combination of CSF tau ratio and mid-saggital midbrain-to-pons atrophy for the early diagnosis of progressive supranu-clear palsy. *J Alzheimers Dis* 2010;22:195-203.

[139] Hampel H, Buerger K, Zinkowski R, et al. Measurement of phosphorylated tau epito-pes in the differential diagnosis of Alzheimer disease: a comparative cerebrospinal fluid study. *Arch Gen Psychiatry* 2004 Jan;61:95-102.

[140] Tang W, Huang Q, Yao YY, Wang Y, Wu YL, Wang ZY. Does CSF p-tau help to discriminate Alzheimer's disease from other dementias and mild cognitive impairment? A meta-analysis of the literature. *J Neural Transm* 2014 May 10.

[141] Hampel H, Blennow K, Shaw LM, Hoessler YC, Zetterberg H, Trojanowski JQ. Total and phosphorylated tau protein as biological markers of Alzheimer's disease. *Exp Gerontol* 2010 Jan;45:30-40.

[142] Sanchez-Juan P, Green A, Ladogana A, et al. CSF tests in the differential diagnosis of Creutzfeldt-Jakob disease. *Neurology* 2006 Aug 22;67:637-643.

[143] Kremer A, Louis JV, Jaworski T, Van LF. GSK3 and Alzheimer's Disease: Facts and Fiction... *Front Mol Neurosci* 2011;4:17.

[144] Llorens F, Zafar S, Ansoleaga B, et al. Subtype and regional regulation of prion biomarkers in sporadic Creutzfeldt-Jakob disease. *Neuropathol Appl Neurobiol* 2014 Aug 18.

[145] Riemenschneider M, Wagenpfeil S, Vanderstichele H, et al. Phospho-tau/total tau ratio in cerebrospinal fluid discriminates Creutzfeldt-Jakob disease from other dementias. *Mol Psychiatry* 2003 Mar;8:343-347.

[146] Schmidt C, Haik S, Satoh K, et al. Rapidly progressive Alzheimer's disease: a multicenter update. *J Alzheimers Dis* 2012;30:751-756.

[147] Kester MI, van der Vlies AE, Blankenstein MA, et al. CSF biomarkers predict rate of cognitive decline in Alzheimer disease. *Neurology* 2009 Oct 27;73:1353-1358.

[148] Visser PJ, Verhey F, Knol DL, et al. Prevalence and prognostic value of CSF markers of Alzheimer's disease pathology in patients with subjective cognitive impairment or mild cognitive impairment in the DESCRIPA study: a prospective cohort study. *Lancet Neurol* 2009 Jul;8:619-627.

[149] Amor S, Peferoen LA, Vogel DY, et al. Inflammation in neurodegenerative diseases--an update. *Immunology* 2014 Jun;142:151-166.

[150] Aguzzi A, Barres BA, Bennett ML. Microglia: scapegoat, saboteur, or something else? *Science* 2013 Jan 11;339:156-161.

[151] Akiyama H, Barger S, Barnum S, et al. Inflammation and Alzheimer's disease. *Neurobiol Aging* 2000 May;21:383-421.

[152] Alcolea D, Carmona-Iragui M, Suarez-Calvet M, et al. Relationship Between beta-Secretase, Inflammation and Core Cerebrospinal Fluid Biomarkers for Alzheimer's Disease. *J Alzheimers Dis* 2014 May 12.

[153] Llorens F, Lopez-Gonzalez I, Thune K, et al. Subtype and regional-specific neuroinflammation in sporadic creutzfeldt-jakob disease. *Front Aging Neurosci* 2014;6:198.

[154] Stoeck K, Bodemer M, Zerr I. Pro- and anti-inflammatory cytokines in the CSF of patients with Creutzfeldt-Jakob disease. *J Neuroimmunol* 2006 Mar;172:175-181.

[155] Stoeck K, Bodemer M, Ciesielczyk B, et al. Interleukin 4 and interleukin 10 levels are elevated in the cerebrospinal fluid of patients with Creutzfeldt-Jakob disease. *Arch Neurol* 2005 Oct;62:1591-1594.

[156] Swardfager W, Lanctot K, Rothenburg L, Wong A, Cappell J, Herrmann N. A meta-analysis of cytokines in Alzheimer's disease. *Biol Psychiatry* 2010 Nov 15;68:930-941.

[157] Rota E, Bellone G, Rocca P, Bergamasco B, Emanuelli G, Ferrero P. Increased intrathecal TGF-beta1, but not IL-12, IFN-gamma and IL-10 levels in Alzheimer's disease patients. *Neurol Sci* 2006 Apr;27:33-39.

[158] Tarkowski E, Andreasen N, Tarkowski A, Blennow K. Intrathecal inflammation precedes development of Alzheimer's disease. *J Neurol Neurosurg Psychiatry* 2003 Sep; 74:1200-1205.

[159] Schuitemaker A, Dik MG, Veerhuis R, et al. Inflammatory markers in AD and MCI patients with different biomarker profiles. *Neurobiol Aging* 2009 Nov;30:1885-1889.

[160] Wang KX, Denhardt DT. Osteopontin: role in immune regulation and stress responses. *Cytokine Growth Factor Rev* 2008 Oct;19:333-345.

[161] Comi C, Carecchio M, Chiocchetti A, et al. Osteopontin is increased in the cerebrospinal fluid of patients with Alzheimer's disease and its levels correlate with cognitive decline. *J Alzheimers Dis* 2010;19:1143-1148.

[162] Sun Y, Yin XS, Guo H, Han RK, He RD, Chi LJ. Elevated osteopontin levels in mild cognitive impairment and Alzheimer's disease. *Mediators Inflamm* 2013;2013:615745.

[163] Bornsen L, Khademi M, Olsson T, Sorensen PS, Sellebjerg F. Osteopontin concentrations are increased in cerebrospinal fluid during attacks of multiple sclerosis. *Mult Scler* 2011 Jan;17:32-42.

[164] Verwey NA, Schuitemaker A, van der Flier WM, et al. Serum amyloid p component as a biomarker in mild cognitive impairment and Alzheimer's disease. *Dement Geriatr Cogn Disord* 2008;26:522-527.

[165] Naude PJ, Nyakas C, Eiden LE, et al. Lipocalin 2: novel component of proinflammatory signaling in Alzheimer's disease. *FASEB J* 2012 Jul;26:2811-2823.

[166] Alcolea D, Carmona-Iragui M, Suarez-Calvet M, et al. Relationship Between beta-Secretase, Inflammation and Core Cerebrospinal Fluid Biomarkers for Alzheimer's Disease. *J Alzheimers Dis* 2014 Jan 1;42:157-167.

[167] Perrin RJ, Craig-Schapiro R, Malone JP, et al. Identification and validation of novel cerebrospinal fluid biomarkers for staging early Alzheimer's disease. *PLoS One* 2011;6:e16032.

[168] Craig-Schapiro R, Perrin RJ, Roe CM, et al. YKL-40: a novel prognostic fluid biomarker for preclinical Alzheimer's disease. *Biol Psychiatry* 2010 Nov 15;68:903-912.

[169] Antonell A, Mansilla A, Rami L, et al. Cerebrospinal Fluid Level of YKL-40 Protein in Preclinical and Prodromal Alzheimer's Disease. *J Alzheimers Dis* 2014 Jul 2.

[170] Krol J, Loedige I, Filipowicz W. The widespread regulation of microRNA biogenesis, function and decay. *Nat Rev Genet* 2010 Sep;11:597-610.

[171] Gascon E, Gao FB. Cause or Effect: Misregulation of microRNA Pathways in Neurodegeneration. *Front Neurosci* 2012;6:48.

[172] Maciotta S, Meregalli M, Torrente Y. The involvement of microRNAs in neurodegenerative diseases. *Front Cell Neurosci* 2013;7:265.

[173] Lehmann SM, Kruger C, Park B, et al. An unconventional role for miRNA: let-7 activates Toll-like receptor 7 and causes neurodegeneration. *Nat Neurosci* 2012 Jun; 15:827-835.

[174] Salta E, De SB. Non-coding RNAs with essential roles in neurodegenerative disorders. *Lancet Neurol* 2012 Feb;11:189-200.

[175] Eacker SM, Dawson TM, Dawson VL. Understanding microRNAs in neurodegeneration. *Nat Rev Neurosci* 2009 Dec;10:837-841.

[176] Cheng L, Quek CY, Sun X, Bellingham SA, Hill AF. The detection of microRNA associated with Alzheimer's disease in biological fluids using next-generation sequencing technologies. *Front Genet* 2013;4:150.

[177] McAlexander MA, Phillips MJ, Witwer KW. Comparison of Methods for miRNA Extraction from Plasma and Quantitative Recovery of RNA from Cerebrospinal Fluid. *Front Genet* 2013;4:83.

[178] Pritchard CC, Cheng HH, Tewari M. MicroRNA profiling: approaches and considerations. *Nat Rev Genet* 2012 May;13:358-369.

[179] Weiland M, Gao XH, Zhou L, Mi QS. Small RNAs have a large impact: circulating microRNAs as biomarkers for human diseases. *RNA Biol* 2012 Jun;9:850-859.

[180] Sala FC, Lau P, Salta E, et al. Reduced expression of hsa-miR-27a-3p in CSF of patients with Alzheimer disease. *Neurology* 2013 Dec 10;81:2103-2106.

[181] Kiko T, Nakagawa K, Tsuduki T, Furukawa K, Arai H, Miyazawa T. MicroRNAs in plasma and cerebrospinal fluid as potential markers for Alzheimer's disease. *J Alzheimers Dis* 2014;39:253-259.

[182] Muller M, Kuiperij HB, Claassen JA, Kusters B, Verbeek MM. MicroRNAs in Alzheimer's disease: differential expression in hippocampus and cell-free cerebrospinal fluid. *Neurobiol Aging* 2014 Jan;35:152-158.

[183] Lukiw WJ, Zhao Y, Cui JG. An NF-kappaB-sensitive micro RNA-146a-mediated inflammatory circuit in Alzheimer disease and in stressed human brain cells. *J Biol Chem* 2008 Nov 14;283:31315-31322.

[184] Lukiw WJ, Dua P, Pogue AI, Eicken C, Hill JM. Upregulation of micro RNA-146a (miRNA-146a), a marker for inflammatory neurodegeneration, in sporadic Creutzfeldt-Jakob disease (sCJD) and Gerstmann-Straussler-Scheinker (GSS) syndrome. *J Toxicol Environ Health A* 2011;74:1460-1468.

[185] Li YY, Cui JG, Hill JM, Bhattacharjee S, Zhao Y, Lukiw WJ. Increased expression of miRNA-146a in Alzheimer's disease transgenic mouse models. *Neurosci Lett* 2011 Jan 3;487:94-98.

[186] Iyer A, Zurolo E, Prabowo A, et al. MicroRNA-146a: a key regulator of astrocyte-mediated inflammatory response. *PLoS One* 2012;7:e44789.

[187] Boldin MP, Taganov KD, Rao DS, et al. miR-146a is a significant brake on autoimmunity, myeloproliferation, and cancer in mice. *J Exp Med* 2011 Jun 6;208:1189-1201.

[188] Podlesniy P, Figueiro-Silva J, Llado A, et al. Low cerebrospinal fluid concentration of mitochondrial DNA in preclinical Alzheimer disease. *Ann Neurol* 2013 Nov; 74:655-668.

[189] Schlotterbeck G, Ross A, Dieterle F, Senn H. Metabolic profiling technologies for biomarker discovery in biomedicine and drug development. *Pharmacogenomics* 2006 Oct; 7:1055-1075.

[190] Czech C, Berndt P, Busch K, et al. Metabolite profiling of Alzheimer's disease cerebrospinal fluid. *PLoS One* 2012;7:e31501.

[191] Trushina E, Dutta T, Persson XM, Mielke MM, Petersen RC. Identification of altered metabolic pathways in plasma and CSF in mild cognitive impairment and Alzheimer's disease using metabolomics. *PLoS One* 2013;8:e63644.

[192] Kaddurah-Daouk R, Zhu H, Sharma S, et al. Alterations in metabolic pathways and networks in Alzheimer's disease. *Transl Psychiatry* 2013;3:e244.

[193] Zetterberg H, Wilson D, Andreasson U, et al. Plasma tau levels in Alzheimer's disease. *Alzheimers Res Ther* 2013;5:9.

[194] Hye A, Lynham S, Thambisetty M, et al. Proteome-based plasma biomarkers for Alzheimer's disease. *Brain* 2006 Nov;129:3042-3050.

[195] Hu WT, Holtzman DM, Fagan AM, et al. Plasma multianalyte profiling in mild cognitive impairment and Alzheimer disease. *Neurology* 2012 Aug 28;79:897-905.

[196] Doecke JD, Laws SM, Faux NG, et al. Blood-based protein biomarkers for diagnosis of Alzheimer disease. *Arch Neurol* 2012 Oct;69:1318-1325.

[197] O'Bryant SE, Xiao G, Barber R, et al. A serum protein-based algorithm for the detection of Alzheimer disease. *Arch Neurol* 2010 Sep;67:1077-1081.

[198] Ray S, Britschgi M, Herbert C, et al. Classification and prediction of clinical Alzheimer's diagnosis based on plasma signaling proteins. *Nat Med* 2007 Nov;13:1359-1362.

[199] Bjorkqvist M, Ohlsson M, Minthon L, Hansson O. Evaluation of a previously suggested plasma biomarker panel to identify Alzheimer's disease. *PLoS One* 2012;7:e29868.

[200] Soares HD, Chen Y, Sabbagh M, Roher A, Schrijvers E, Breteler M. Identifying early markers of Alzheimer's disease using quantitative multiplex proteomic immunoassay panels. *Ann N Y Acad Sci* 2009 Oct;1180:56-67.

[201] Nagele E, Han M, Demarshall C, Belinka B, Nagele R. Diagnosis of Alzheimer's disease based on disease-specific autoantibody profiles in human sera. *PLoS One* 2011;6:e23112.

[202] Burgos K, Malenica I, Metpally R, et al. Profiles of extracellular miRNA in cerebrospinal fluid and serum from patients with Alzheimer's and Parkinson's diseases correlate with disease status and features of pathology. *PLoS One* 2014;9:e94839.

[203] Galimberti D, Villa C, Fenoglio C, et al. Circulating miRNAs as Potential Biomarkers in Alzheimer's Disease. *J Alzheimers Dis* 2014 Jul 7.

[204] Tan L, Yu JT, Liu QY, et al. Circulating miR-125b as a biomarker of Alzheimer's disease. *J Neurol Sci* 2014 Jan 15;336:52-56.

[205] Tan L, Yu JT, Tan MS, et al. Genome-wide serum microRNA expression profiling identifies serum biomarkers for Alzheimer's disease. *J Alzheimers Dis* 2014;40:1017-1027.

[206] Wang Q, Li P, Li A, et al. Plasma specific miRNAs as predictive biomarkers for diagnosis and prognosis of glioma. *J Exp Clin Cancer Res* 2012;31:97.

[207] Leidinger P, Backes C, Deutscher S, et al. A blood based 12-miRNA signature of Alzheimer disease patients. *Genome Biol* 2013;14:R78.

[208] Schipper HM, Maes OC, Chertkow HM, Wang E. MicroRNA expression in Alzheimer blood mononuclear cells. *Gene Regul Syst Bio* 2007;1:263-274.

[209] Hampel H, Lista S, Teipel SJ, et al. Perspective on future role of biological markers in clinical therapy trials of Alzheimer's disease: a long-range point of view beyond 2020. *Biochem Pharmacol* 2014 Apr 15;88:426-449.

[210] Hampel H, Frank R, Broich K, et al. Biomarkers for Alzheimer's disease: academic, industry and regulatory perspectives. *Nat Rev Drug Discov* 2010 Jul;9:560-574.

[211] Vos SJ, Xiong C, Visser PJ, et al. Preclinical Alzheimer's disease and its outcome: a longitudinal cohort study. *Lancet Neurol* 2013 Oct;12:957-965.

[212] Bateman RJ, Xiong C, Benzinger TL, et al. Clinical and biomarker changes in dominantly inherited Alzheimer's disease. *N Engl J Med* 2012 Aug 30;367:795-804.

[213] Jack CR, Jr., Knopman DS, Jagust WJ, et al. Hypothetical model of dynamic biomarkers of the Alzheimer's pathological cascade. Lancet Neurol 2010 Jan;9:119-128.

[214] Jack CR, Jr., Knopman DS, Jagust WJ, et al. Tracking pathophysiological processes in Alzheimer's disease: an updated hypothetical model of dynamic biomarkers. Lancet Neurol 2013 Feb;12:207-216.

Permissions

All chapters in this book were first published in AD, by InTech Open; hereby published with permission under the Creative Commons Attribution License or equivalent. Every chapter published in this book has been scrutinized by our experts. Their significance has been extensively debated. The topics covered herein carry significant findings which will fuel the growth of the discipline. They may even be implemented as practical applications or may be referred to as a beginning point for another development.

The contributors of this book come from diverse backgrounds, making this book a truly international effort. This book will bring forth new frontiers with its revolutionizing research information and detailed analysis of the nascent developments around the world.

We would like to thank all the contributing authors for lending their expertise to make the book truly unique. They have played a crucial role in the development of this book. Without their invaluable contributions this book wouldn't have been possible. They have made vital efforts to compile up to date information on the varied aspects of this subject to make this book a valuable addition to the collection of many professionals and students.

This book was conceptualized with the vision of imparting up-to-date information and advanced data in this field. To ensure the same, a matchless editorial board was set up. Every individual on the board went through rigorous rounds of assessment to prove their worth. After which they invested a large part of their time researching and compiling the most relevant data for our readers.

The editorial board has been involved in producing this book since its inception. They have spent rigorous hours researching and exploring the diverse topics which have resulted in the successful publishing of this book. They have passed on their knowledge of decades through this book. To expedite this challenging task, the publisher supported the team at every step. A small team of assistant editors was also appointed to further simplify the editing procedure and attain best results for the readers.

Apart from the editorial board, the designing team has also invested a significant amount of their time in understanding the subject and creating the most relevant covers. They scrutinized every image to scout for the most suitable representation of the subject and create an appropriate cover for the book.

The publishing team has been an ardent support to the editorial, designing and production team. Their endless efforts to recruit the best for this project, has resulted in the accomplishment of this book. They are a veteran in the field of academics and their pool of knowledge is as vast as their experience in printing. Their expertise and guidance has proved useful at every step. Their uncompromising quality standards have made this book an exceptional effort. Their encouragement from time to time has been an inspiration for everyone.

The publisher and the editorial board hope that this book will prove to be a valuable piece of knowledge for researchers, students, practitioners and scholars across the globe.

List of Contributors

De Breucker Sandra and Pepersack Thierry
Erasme University Hospital– Free University of Brussels, Department of Geriatrics, Brussels, Belgium

Bier Jean-Christophe
Erasme University Hospital– Free University of Brussels, Department of Neurology, Brussels

Sophie Stukas, Iva Kulic, Shahab Zareyan and Cheryl L. Wellington
Department of Pathology and Laboratory Medicine, Djavad Mowafaghian Centre for Brain Health, University of British Columbia, Vancouver, British Columbia, Canada

Aysegul Uludag, Sibel Cevizci and Ahmet Uludag
Canakkale Onsekiz Mart University, Faculty of Medicine, Department of Family Medicine, Canakkale, Turkey

Francois Bernier, Yoshiaki Sato and Yoshiya Oda
Eisai Co., Ltd., Tokodai, Tsukuba, Ibaraki, Japan

Pavan Kumar
Eisai IncAndover, MA, USA

Miguel Angel Ontiveros Torres, Amparo Viramontes-Pintos and José Luna-Muñoz
Brain Bank-LaNSE CINVESTAV-IPN, Mexico

Luis Oskar Soto-Rojas
Brain Bank-LaNSE CINVESTAV-IPN, Mexico
Departments of Physiology. ENCB IPN, México
FES Iztacala. UNAM, México

Fidel de la Cruz-López
Departments of Physiology. ENCB IPN, México

Citlaltepetl Salinas-Lara
FES Iztacala. UNAM, México
INNN MVS, Mexico

María del Carmen Cárdenas-Aguayo and Marco A. Meraz-Ríos
Molecular Biomedicine Department, CINVESTAV-IPN, Mexico

Benjamín Florán-Garduño
Physiology, Biophysics and Neurosciences Department, CINVESTAV-IPN, Mexico

Sabine Nuhn, Christoph Peter and Katharina Stoeck
Department of Neurology, Clinical Dementia Center, University Medical School, Georg- August University, Göttingen, Germany

Inga Zerr and Franc Llorens
Department of Neurology, Clinical Dementia Center, University Medical School, Georg- August University, Göttingen, Germany
German Center for Neurodegenerative Diseases (DZNE) – Göttingen, Germany

Index

Neuronal Loss, 2, 24-25, 115, 123, 127, 145, 148
Neurotoxicity, 21, 45, 111, 118, 130, 133, 162
Nucleic Acid, 87, 92

O
Occupational Therapy, 69
Oligodendrocytes, 19

P
Phosphatidylcholine, 15, 33
Phosphatidylethanolamine, 15, 20
Polyadenylation, 92
Protofibrils, 78-79, 101

R
Rheumatoid Arthritis, 97

S
Senile Plaques, 2, 115, 128, 147-148, 164
Sphingomyelin, 15, 18, 39, 85
Syncope, 5, 59-61, 73
Syphilis, 2

T
Tau Protein, 2, 72, 79, 100, 110-111, 113-115, 124, 127-128, 146, 149, 162, 166-167
Trypsin, 84

U
Urinary Tract Infection, 5

V
Vascular Dysfunction, 2, 20
Vascular Endothelial Health, 25

www.ingramcontent.com/pod-product-compliance
Lightning Source LLC
Chambersburg PA
CBHW070155240326
41458CB00126B/5241